Preface

High blood pressure is common in the UK. It is a major risk factor for cardiovascular disease and premature death. Reducing the average salt intake of the population is likely to decrease the burden of high blood pressure and improve public health.

Sodium is an essential nutrient and salt is the major source of sodium in the UK diet. Most people, however, consume more sodium than is required. The latest available data show that habitual levels of salt intake are high for both adults and children. For adults, average intake is two and a half times the reference nutrient intake for sodium. Although accurate data are not available for children, conservative estimates indicate that, on a body weight basis, the average salt intake of children is higher than that of adults.

In 1994, the Committee on Medical Aspects of Food and Nutrition Policy (COMA), in a review of nutritional aspects of cardiovascular disease, made a recommendation to reduce the average salt intake of the population from 9g/day to 6g/day which has also been endorsed by the Chief Medical Officer of England. The present report has been prepared in response to a request, from the Food Standards Agency and the Chief Medical Officer of Wales, for a risk assessment of salt by the Scientific Advisory Committee on Nutrition (SACN). The evidence published since 1994 has been appraised, in a methodological fashion, to assess whether the previous recommendation to reduce salt intakes in the population remains valid. It is the first time that an expert committee has specifically undertaken a review of the evidence on salt and health in the UK.

There is now a larger body of evidence, which draws an association between salt consumption and blood pressure. SACN has concluded that the habitual salt intake of the population raises the risk of high blood pressure, which in turn increases the risk of stroke and premature death from cardiovascular diseases. The risk increases with age and is not simply a feature of those with the highest salt intakes or the highest levels of blood pressure but graded and evident across a range of salt intakes that are habitual in the UK.

The report accepts the previous recommendation for a reduction in the population average intake of salt to 6g per day for adults and for the first time has set targets for children which are proportionate to their needs. Meeting these targets would be of major benefit to public health. Even a small reduction in salt intake could help to reduce the burden of high blood pressure in our population.

A public health approach to reducing salt levels is required. A targeted approach to salt reduction by health professionals dealing with patients with diagnosed hypertension, by itself, may not be enough.

The draft of this report was made available for comment and I thank all those who responded. The comments were carefully considered during finalisation of the report. The responsibility of SACN is for an assessment of risk. Many of the comments received during the consultation related to the management or communication of risk, and hence were outside the remit of the committee.

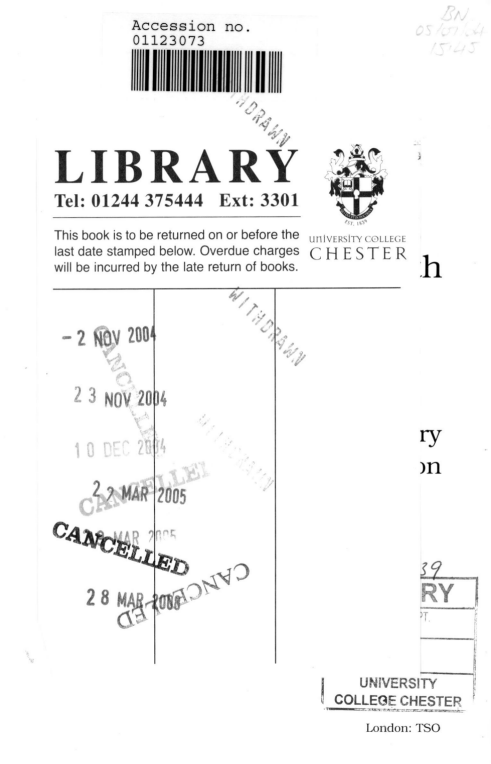
London: TSO

It is for the Government to consider the action required to achieve the recommended reductions in the salt intake of the population. Achieving these targets will not be easy, as a substantial reduction in salt intake is required. This will entail a sustained, gradual reduction in the salt content of food over a number of years.

Most salt in the diet does not come from addition to food in the home by consumers but from processed foods. This makes it extremely difficult for individuals to reduce their own salt intake and to maintain a reduced intake over any length of time. Key to achieving a sustained salt reduction for public health benefit is the engagement of the food industry (manufacturers, retailers and caterers). All consumers, including children, need more information on salt and sodium, particularly on the adverse health effects of excessive salt consumption, to enable them to make healthy dietary choices and reduce salt in their diet.

The Committee also identified the need for improving the existing evidence base, which might facilitate salt reduction strategies, particularly on:

- how patterns of salt intake vary across and within groups of the population;

- the contribution home prepared meals and foods eaten outside the home make to overall salt intakes in the UK;

- the processing techniques and new technologies that can help to reduce salt content of foods whilst maintaining safety and palatability.

The potential public health rewards of salt reduction at a population level through lowering the salt content of manufactured foods has international support. There is compelling evidence that this is an effective and appropriate means to reduce the public health burden of cardiovascular disease to society and the risk of ill health to individuals.

Professor Alan Jackson
Chair of the Scientific Advisory Committee on Nutrition

April 2003

Contents

Membership of Scientific Advisory Committee on Nutrition: Salt Subgroup

Chairman

Professor Alan Jackson   Professor of Human Nutrition, School of Medicine, University of Southampton

Members

Professor Peter Aggett   Professor of Child Health. Head of School, Lancashire Postgraduate School of Medicine and Health

Miss Gill Fine   Head of Food and Health, Sainsbury's Supermarkets Ltd

Professor Sheila Bingham   Deputy Director, Dunn Human Nutrition Unit, Medical Research Council

Secretariat for Salt Subgroup

Food Standards Agency
Dr Lisa Jackson (Medical) (Until November '02)
Dr Alison Tedstone (Scientific)
Ms Mamta Singh (Scientific)
Dr Tracey Dean (Scientific) (Until November '01)

Department of Health
Dr Sheela Reddy (Scientific)
Dr Adrienne Cullum (Scientific)

Membership of Scientific Advisory Committee on Nutrition

Chairman

Professor Alan Jackson | Professor of Human Nutrition, School of Medicine, University of Southampton

Members

Professor Peter Aggett | Head of School, Lancashire Postgraduate School of Medicine and Health, Professor of Child Health and Nutrition University of Lancashire

Professor Annie Anderson | Research Professor of Food Choice, Centre for Public Health Nutrition Research, Ninewells Medical School, University of Dundee

Professor Sheila Bingham | Deputy Director, Medical Research Council's Dunn Human Nutrition Research, Cambridge

Professor John Cummings | Professor of Experimental Gastroenterology, Department of Molecular and Cellular Pathology, University of Dundee

Miss Gillian Fine | Head of Food and Health, Sainsbury's Supermarkets Ltd

Ms Paulette Jones (Until September '02)	Senior Mentoring Development Officer, DIVERT Trust (The National Charity for the Prevention of Youth Crime), London
Dr Tim Key	Reader in Epidemiology, University of Oxford ICRF Cancer Epidemiology Unit, Radcliffe Infirmary, Oxford
Professor Peter Kopelman	Professor of Clinical Medicine Deputy Warden, Barts and The London, Queen Mary's School of Medicine and Dentistry, University of London
Dr Ann Prentice	Director, Medical Research Council's Dunn Human Nutrition Research,
Professor Emeritus Andrew Rugg-Gunn	Retired Clinical Professor, Newcastle University and Newcastle NHS Trust
Dr Anita Thomas	Consultant Physician, General (Internal) and Geriatric Medicine, Derriford Hospital, Plymouth
Mrs Stella Walsh	Senior Lecturer, Leeds Metropolitan University. National Federation of Consumer Groups
Dr Anthony Williams	Senior Lecturer & Consultant, Neonatal Paediatrics, St. George's Hospital, London
Professor Christine Williams	Professor of Human Nutrition, University of Reading

Observers

Mr Tom Murray	Food Standards Agency
Ms Imogen Sharp	Department of Health
Dr Martin Donaghy (until December '02)	Scottish Executive Health Department
Dr Barbara Davis (from January '03)	Scottish Executive Health Department
Mrs Maureen Howell	The Welsh Assembly, Health Promotion Division
Dr Elizabeth Mitchell	Department of Health, Social Sciences and Public Safety, Northern Ireland
Ms Danila Armstrong	Department of Health

Secretariat

Food Standards Agency
Dr Lisa Jackson (Medical) (Until November '02))
Dr Alison Tedstone (Scientific)
Mr Ben Walters (Administrative)
Mr Jeff Allder (Administrative)
Ms Orla Yeates (Administrative) (Until August '02))

Department of Health
Dr Sheela Reddy (Scientific)
Dr Adrienne Cullum (Scientific)
Mr Fayaz Aziz (Administrative) (Until October '02)

Summary

Background

Increased blood pressure, or hypertension, is the most common outcome that has been associated with high levels of salt intake. Hypertension is a major risk factor in the development of cardiovascular disease. The relative risk of cardiovascular disease increases as blood pressure rises even within what is considered the normal range of blood pressure, indicating that large numbers of people are at risk.

Although the key evidence for the association between high salt intakes and blood pressure relates to sodium, the major dietary source of sodium is salt. The relationship between salt and blood pressure was previously considered in 1994 by the Committee on Medical Aspects of Food and Nutrition Policy (COMA) as part of their report on *Nutritional Aspects of Cardiovascular Disease*. COMA recommended a reduction in the average intake of salt by the adult population from 9g to 6g per day. A similar proportionate reduction in the salt content of children's diets was recommended, but insufficient data were available to enable quantification.

The Scientific Advisory Committee on Nutrition (SACN) was asked by the Food Standards Agency and the Chief Medical Officer of Wales to review the evidence since 1994 and to consider making recommendations for children.

Methodology

The key issues for consideration were: physiological requirements for sodium; salt sensitivity; effects of salt on blood pressure; and morbidity and premature mortality outcomes. The framework for risk assessment developed by SACN (2002), was used as a template to identify and evaluate the available evidence.

Main findings

Physiological requirements for sodium:

• No basis was found for a revision of the 1991 Dietary Reference Values for sodium or to change the 1994 COMA recommendation for a target salt intake of 6g/day (2.4g/100 mmol sodium) for the adult population. 6g is higher than the Reference Nutrient Intake (RNI) and substantially greater than the salt intake required to maintain the sodium content of the body.

• The RNI values previously agreed by COMA (1991) for infants and children were accepted and used as a basis to set the daily target average salt intakes. These were: less than 1g/day for 0-6m; 1g/day for 7-12m; 2g/day for 1-3y; 3g/day for 4-6y; 5g/day for 7-10y; 6g/day for 11-14y.

• The target salt intakes set for adults and children do not represent ideal or optimum consumption levels, but achievable population goals.

Salt sensitivity

• There is no agreed definition or clinical criteria to identify salt sensitivity. The greatest benefits are likely to be achieved by taking a population approach to reducing salt intakes, rather than through individual targeted advice.

Effects of salt on blood pressure

- Since 1994, the evidence of an association between dietary salt intakes and blood pressure has increased. The data have been consistent in various study populations and across the age range in adults.

- The greatest reductions in blood pressure are observed when a diet rich in fruits, vegetables, and low-fat dairy foods, and reduced in saturated and total fat, is combined with a low salt diet.

- Long-term effects of dietary advice to reduce dietary salt levels show that significant effects of salt reduction on lowering blood pressure at 6 months are not sustained over time. This reflects the difficulties faced by individuals in lowering salt intake, as most dietary salt originates from processed food.

Morbidity and premature mortality outcomes

- There are insufficient reliable data on long-term effects of salt on cardiovascular disease outcomes to reach clear conclusions.

- Evidence suggests that high salt intake causes left ventricular hypertrophy, a strong risk factor for cardiovascular disease, independently of blood pressure effects.

- While high salt intakes have been associated with detrimental effects on bone health, there are insufficient data to draw firm conclusions.

Children

- There is a lack of data for effects of salt intake in childhood on cardiovascular health.

- Data on the contribution of dietary salt to raised blood pressure in children is limited and it is unclear whether sodium intake in isolation is a factor in the development of hypertension in the young which then tracks into adulthood.

- The evidence suggests long-term consumption of salt by children at levels currently habitual for adults being potentially harmful in later life; it would therefore be inadvisable for children to become accustomed to this level of consumption.

Conclusions

- Reducing the average population salt intake would proportionally lower population average blood pressure levels and confer significant public health benefits by contributing to a reduction in the burden of cardiovascular disease.

- To achieve the recommended levels of salt intake for adults and children, a substantial reduction in the current average salt intake of the population is required. This would be best achieved using a population-based approach through the adoption of a healthy balanced diet, which is low in salt and saturated and total fat, and rich in fruit, vegetables, and complex carbohydrates.

- A reduction in the salt content of processed food and drinks is necessary which requires the continued co-operation of food manufacturers, retailers, and caterers.

1 Scientific Advisory Committee on Nutrition: Salt and Health

Background

1.1 High levels of salt intake have been associated with raised blood pressure, also known as hypertension.

1.2 The relationship between salt and blood pressure was previously considered by the Committee on Medical Aspects of Food and Nutrition Policy (COMA) in 1994, which recommended a target for reduction in the population average intakes of salt to 6g per day for adults (DH[1], 1994). The Government continues to receive representations from interested parties regarding the extent to which the evidence since 1994, on salt intake and health, has been appraised.

Terms of reference

1.3 In September 2001, the Scientific Advisory Committee on Nutrition (SACN[2]) was asked by the Food Standards Agency, supported by the Chief Medical Officer (CMO) of Wales, to:

- review the evidence since the 1994 COMA recommendations on salt intake, taking into account the submissions that had been received from interested parties;

- consider making recommendations for children.

1 Department of Health
2 SACN succeeded COMA in 2001

1.4   A *Salt Subgroup*, comprising members from SACN, was established to take this work forward.

Methodology

1.5   Taking account of submissions received from interested parties (listed in Annex 1), key issues for consideration were identified. These were: physiological requirements for sodium; salt sensitivity; effects of salt on blood pressure; and morbidity and premature mortality outcomes.

1.6   The framework for risk assessment developed by SACN (2002), which recognises the contribution of different types of studies in providing different kinds of information, was used as a template to identify and evaluate the available evidence since 1994. Evidence from different types of studies was considered in order to make an overall assessment. For example, long-term studies provide information about compliance, effectiveness, and adaptive responses to changes in dietary intake; short-term studies are useful for assessing physiological responses; whilst animal data are helpful for examining possible mechanisms and enable dose response evaluations.

1.7   Greater weight was placed on studies that had determined sodium intake by measuring sodium excretion from 24-hour urine collections, as this is the most accurate way to assess salt intake. Dietary intake methods could not be considered as reliable since salt added during cooking or at the table is not always taken into account, and because of measurement errors associated with these methods.

1.8   Most of the recent published evidence regarding physiological requirements for sodium related to high intakes, with few data available on low intakes. It was therefore necessary to refer to studies published before 1994 for consideration of a minimum safe intake.

1.9   The information sources and search terms used for identifying relevant studies, the full list of studies that were examined, and the procedures for finalisation of the report, can be found in Annex 2.

2 Introduction

2.1   The key evidence for the association between high dietary intakes of salt and blood pressure relates to sodium. The major source of sodium in the diet is from salt (sodium chloride); therefore, in practical terms, any recommendation for sodium reduction will translate into salt reduction. The terms salt and sodium are often used synonymously, however, on a weight basis, salt comprises 40% sodium and 60% chloride[3].

Dietary exposure to salt

2.2   Sodium is present in plant and animal derived foods as well as drinking water. As salt, it is added to foods during processing, cooking, and at the table. The main reasons for addition of salt in food manufacture are for flavour, texture and preservation. Major dietary sources of sodium are from salt added during the processing and manufacture of foods (non-discretionary) and salt added to food during cooking and at the table (discretionary).

2.3   It is estimated that about 15-20% of total dietary sodium intake is from discretionary sources. Naturally occurring sodium in unprocessed foods contributes approximately 15% of total sodium intake. Therefore manufactured foods contribute about 65-70% of dietary sodium (British Nutrition Foundation, 1994).

2.4   The main sources of sodium from foods and the contribution of each to the salt intake for adults and children are listed in Annex 3. Cereals and cereal products

---

3 1g of sodium is equivalent to 2.55g salt (2.5g is used by industry for labelling purposes); 1 mmol sodium is equivalent to 23mg sodium.

(which include bread, breakfast cereals, biscuits, cakes and pastries) provide nearly 40% of average intake, and meat and meat products contribute approximately 21% to average intake.

2.5   Assessments of patterns of salt consumption by population groups or individuals over time are not available. The National Food Survey (NFS) does however provide information on household food consumption. A comparison of the 1994 NFS (MAFF[4], 1995) and the 2000 NFS (DEFRA[5], 2001) shows that the contribution made by processed foods to the total household intake of salt was 83% in 1995 and 86% in 2000. There are no robust data on the amount of salt consumed outside the home, but this could be substantial for some groups.

2.6   The most accurate method to determine salt intake (dietary exposure) is from complete 24-hour urine collections. Measurement of intake from dietary assessment methods alone is considered unreliable. For adults, Gregory et al (1990) found that assessment from food records, compared to measurements from 24-hour urine collections, underestimated salt intakes by 19%. Although salt intake is more accurately measured using 24-hour urine collections, even these do not measure absolute amounts unless results have been corrected using a marker for completeness of collections (Bingham & Cummings, 1985; Bingham et al, 1988).

2.7   Three national dietary surveys provide information on the salt intakes of the UK population: the 1987 Dietary and Nutritional Survey of British adults (Gregory et al, 1990); the 1997 National Diet and Nutrition Survey (NDNS) of young

4 Ministry of Agriculture, Fisheries & Food.
5 Department of Environment, Food & Rural Affairs.

people (Gregory et al, 2000); and the 1994/5 NDNS of people aged 65 and over (Finch et al, 1998).

2.8 The adult survey (Gregory et al, 1990), which utilised 24-hour urine collections, reported an average daily salt intake of 9g (3.6g/150 mmol sodium). Average sodium excretion for men was 173 mmol (4.2g sodium/10.4g salt) and 132 mmol (3.2g sodium/7.9g salt) for women.

2.9 The 1997 NDNS of young people (Gregory et al, 2000), based on dietary intake, provides data on average salt intakes for 4-18 year-olds which are set out in Table 1.

Table 1: NDNS data on average daily sodium intakes from food consumed by young people (4-18yrs)

Age (years)	Male		Female	
	Sodium	Estimated Salt	Sodium	Estimated Salt
	g/d (mmol/d)	g/d	g/d (mmol/d)	g/d
4-6	2.07 (90)	5.3	1.86 (81)	4.7
7-10	2.40 (105)	6.1	2.16 (94)	5.5
11-14	2.70 (118)	6.9	2.27 (99)	5.8
15-18	3.30 (142)	8.3	2.28 (99)	5.8

2.10 The 1994/5 NDNS (Finch et al, 1998), also based on dietary assessment, showed average salt intakes from food for people aged 65 years and over were 6.8g/day (2.7g/ 117 mmol sodium) for men and 5.3g/day (2.1g/91 mmol sodium) for women.

2.11 The 1994/5 and 1997 surveys did not collect 24-hour urine. Dietary methods were used to assess salt intake and salt added to food during cooking or at the table was not included. Consequently, the salt intakes reported are almost certainly underestimates of the actual amounts consumed.

Current recommendations

2.12 In their report on *Dietary Reference Values* (DH, 1991), for ages 15 years upwards, COMA set a lower reference nutrient intake (LRNI[6]) of 0.6g/24 mmol sodium (1.4g salt) per day and a reference nutrient intake (RNI[7]) of 1.6g/70 mmol sodium (4g salt) per day. (See Annex 4 for full range of Dietary Reference Values for sodium across the different age bands.)

2.13 The relationship between salt and blood pressure was more extensively considered in COMA's subsequent report, *Nutritional Aspects of Cardiovascular Disease* (DH, 1994). It was concluded that salt intake is an important determinant of high blood pressure in the population as a whole, in part by influencing the rise of blood pressure with age.

2.14 COMA recommended a reduction in the average intake of salt by the adult population from 9g/day (3.6g/150 mmol sodium), the level current at the time, to 6g/day (2.4g/100 mmol/sodium). Adjusting for the different caloric intakes, this amount represents 5g/day (2g/85 mmol sodium) for women and 7g/day (2.7g/115 mmol sodium) for men. A similar proportionate reduction in the salt content of children's diets was recommended, but insufficient data were available to enable quantification.

6 The LRNI represents the amount of a nutrient likely to meet the needs of 2.5% of the population.
7 The RNI represents the amount of a nutrient likely to meet the needs of 97.5% of the population.

2.15   The target reduction in average salt intake recommended by COMA, from 9g (3.6g/150 mmol sodium) to 6g (2.4g/100 mmol sodium) per day, was considered to be an achievable goal for the UK population rather than an optimal or ideal level of consumption. COMA agreed that a reduction of salt intake to this level would be of demonstrable benefit to the population (DH, 1994).

Current Government position

2.16   The CMO of England has endorsed the 1994 COMA recommendation for a reduction in adult salt consumption to 6g per day (2.4g/100 mmol sodium) (DH, 2001). The COMA recommendation is also advocated by Health Departments in Wales and Northern Ireland. The *Diet Action Plan for Scotland* (Scottish Executive, 1996) has set a target for reduction in average intakes of salt from 9.6g per day (163 mmol/3.8g sodium) to 6g per day (2.4g/100 mmol sodium) by the year 2005.

2.17   The Government accepts that there is a large body of authoritative opinion favouring a general reduction in salt consumption. It is actively engaged in discussions with the food industry, including the retail, manufacturing and catering sectors, regarding ways to broaden public choice in, and reduce the salt content of, processed foods and meals/foods available at catering outlets.

Current initiatives to reduce the salt content of processed foods

2.18   The scope for reducing the salt content of foods is influenced by several factors such as palatability, consumer acceptance, and safety. In recent years, some food manufacturers and retailers have reported significant reductions in the salt content of certain products (Wheelock & Hobbiss, 1999), by gradually adjusting levels over time so that changes in taste are imperceptible. The extent to which the catering industry has moved towards this goal is unknown.

2.19   Low salt and lower salt options of standard products have also become available to help broaden choice. Preference for these products is variable, as is consumer understanding of the role of salt in health.

2.20   Several food manufacturers and retailers have helped improve consumer understanding about the salt content of foods by developing Guideline Daily Amounts (GDAs[8]) for use on food labels and in leaflets. The GDAs of 5g for women and 7g for men are based on the COMA dietary recommendations. In addition, the sodium figure provided in the nutrition panel is converted by several retailers and manufacturers into a salt value to make it easier for the consumer to assess the contribution that the food makes to their overall intake.

8 GDAs are based on the predicted daily consumption by an average adult consumer eating a diet conforming to COMA recommendations. They are not targets for individuals but are guidelines which provide consumers with information to improve understanding of daily consumption of calories, total fat and saturated fats. Some retailers also include information on salt.

3 Public Health Issues

Blood pressure

3.1 Blood is pumped around the body by the left ventricle of the heart imparting a pressure that is opposed by the resistance of the blood vessels through which it flows. The balance of these two opposing forces produces blood pressure. The blood pressure in the major arteries rises and falls as the heart contracts and relaxes. The peak, when the heart contracts, is known as the systolic pressure and the minimum, when the heart relaxes, as diastolic pressure. Blood pressure is measured in terms of the height (millimetres) of a column of mercury (Hg) which it can support and is conventionally recorded as systolic pressure over diastolic pressure, e.g. 120/80 millimetres of mercury (mm Hg).

3.2 Blood pressure must be maintained within certain limits. It needs to be high enough to ensure adequate blood flow to the brain and other tissues, but not so high as to create extra work for the heart and risk damage to the heart and blood vessels.

Hypertension

3.3 High blood pressure (both systolic and diastolic), known as hypertension, is an important risk factor for cardiovascular disease (MacMahon et al, 1990). The CMO of England, in his Annual Report (DH, 2001), highlighted that people with high blood pressure are three times more likely to develop heart disease and stroke, and twice as likely to die from these diseases than those with normal levels. High blood pressure is both a certified cause of death and a contributory factor in over 170,000 deaths per year in England alone.

3.4 There are two clinical classifications of hypertension. Primary (essential) hypertension is of unknown cause and is responsible for at least 90% of cases. In secondary hypertension a recognised medical condition, such as kidney disease, can be ascertained.

3.5 *British Hypertension Society Guidelines* (Ramsay et al, 1999) identify important lifestyle factors that contribute to hypertension as: high salt intake; being overweight; physical inactivity; and excess alcohol consumption.

3.6 A relationship between salt intake and high blood pressure has previously been acknowledged by COMA (DH, 1994). Primary hypertension is the most common outcome that has been associated with high levels of salt intake.

3.7 During the late 1990s the threshold for defining hypertension was lowered, from 160 mm Hg systolic and 95 mm Hg diastolic, to 140 mm Hg systolic and 90 mm Hg diastolic. This reflects observations from clinical trials of blood pressure control for the reduction of major cardiovascular events (Ramsay et al, 1999).

3.8 Cut-off points for the definition of hypertension are useful for clinical purposes, enabling decisions to be made regarding pragmatic thresholds for treatment, however they do not reflect the continuous nature of the relationship between blood pressure and health outcomes. The relative risk for cardiovascular disease increases even within what is considered the normal blood pressure range (both systolic and diastolic), signifying large numbers of people are at risk (Stamler et al, 1993).

3.9   The continuous nature of the risk throughout the accepted normal range of usual blood pressure was confirmed by a meta-analysis of 61 prospective studies of blood pressure and mortality, which obtained data for one million adults with no previous vascular disease at baseline (Prospective Studies Collaboration, 2002). The analyses related the risk of death during five decades of age (40-89y) to the estimated usual systolic and diastolic blood pressure levels at the start of that decade. Usual blood pressure, from as low as 115/ 75 mm Hg, was positively associated with the risk of death from vascular disease.

Prevalence of hypertension in the UK

3.10   Blood pressure levels in the UK rise with age, but this phenomenon is not observed in all populations (Intersalt Cooperative Research Group, 1988) and thus is not an inevitable consequence of ageing. Mean population blood pressures for England, Scotland and Northern Ireland are given in Annex 5 (data for Wales were not available).

3.11   The 2001 Health Survey for **England** (Bajekal et al, 2003) reported that the prevalence of high blood pressure (defined as equal to or greater than 140/90 mm Hg) was 41% for men and 35% for women. The prevalence increased with age from 20% in men aged 16-24 years to 70% in those aged 75 and over; for women, the corresponding rise was from 6% to 79%.

3.12   In **Scotland**, the Scottish Health Survey 1998 (Scottish Executive Health Department, 2000) reported an overall prevalence for hypertension (defined as blood pressure equal to or greater than 140/90 mm Hg) of 33% for men and

28% for women. The prevalence increased from 10% in men aged 16-24 to 74% in those aged 65-74 years. In the same age groups for women, the prevalence increased from 4% to 76%.

3.13   The available data for Wales and Northern Ireland are not comparable with that for England and Scotland, as they are not based on direct blood pressure measurements. In **Wales**, the Welsh Health Survey 1998 (National Assembly for Wales, 1999) showed the proportion of people that reported they had received treatment for raised blood pressure was 14% in 1995 and 15% in 1998. In **Northern Ireland**, the Northern Ireland Health and Social Wellbeing Survey (DHSSPS NI[9], 2001) reported that 19% of men and 27% of women had been informed by a health professional that they had high blood pressure; the prevalence of diagnosed high blood pressure increased with age for both sexes.

Population approach to blood pressure reduction

3.14   A population-based approach to public health is directed at an entire population, rather than those individuals perceived to be at high-risk, in order to address risks that are widespread throughout the population. Such a strategy is based on the observation that a small reduction in risk of a large number of people may result in a large reduction in risk of an entire population (Rose, 1992).

3.15   The risk from cardiovascular disease associated with high blood pressure is not confined to those who are considered hypertensive, but includes large numbers of people in the usual blood pressure range (Prospective Studies

9 Department of Health, Social Services and Public Safety, Northern Ireland.

Collaboration, 2002). Furthermore, the 2001 Health Survey for England (Bajekal et al, 2003) revealed that 66% of adults with hypertension were not in receipt of any treatment. This suggests that the population as a whole may be at a relatively high risk of premature mortality and confirms that population-wide preventive measures to reduce blood pressure are warranted. Such measures should cause a downward shift in the population distribution of blood pressure, which would also benefit high-risk groups.

3.16   On a population basis it has been estimated that a reduction of 2 mm Hg in diastolic blood pressure would result in 15% reduction in risk of stroke and transient ischaemic attacks, and a 6% reduction in risk of coronary heart disease (Cook et al, 1995). McPherson et al (2002) have estimated that 6% of deaths from coronary heart disease could be avoided if the numbers of people with high blood pressure were reduced by 50%.

Other outcomes

3.17   There is some evidence that high intakes of salt may be linked to cardiovascular outcomes independent of blood pressure, such as left ventricular hypertrophy. Very high intakes have been associated with gastric cancer, but the evidence does not generally relate to foods typically consumed in the UK (DH, 1998). There have also been suggestions of an association between salt consumption and the risk of osteoporosis. Although this report focuses primarily on the evidence in relation to hypertension, some discussion of evidence in relation to other health outcomes and premature mortality is included.

4 Review of the Evidence Since 1994

4.1 Evidence for a role of salt in hypertension comes from epidemiological studies between and within populations, controlled clinical trials in normotensive and hypertensive populations, physiological studies, and research in experimental models, including primates.

Physiological requirements for sodium

4.2 Sodium is a vital constituent of the body and thus is an essential nutrient. It is the principal cation in the extracellular fluid (ECF) and plays a key role in maintaining the water balance of the body. It is essential for the maintenance of ECF volume, ECF oncotic pressure, acid-base balance, and muscle and nerve activity. It is also required for the generation of transmembrane gradients, which enable energy dependent uptake of nutrients by the cell, including those of the intestinal mucosa and renal tubules. All of the functions of sodium are interdependent with potassium.

4.3 Sodium balance is interlinked with the maintenance of water homeostasis, which in turn depends on the regulation of ECF volume. A decrease in ECF volume, caused by decreasing plasma volume, leads to a decrease in blood pressure. Conversely, an increase in ECF volume increases blood pressure by increasing plasma volume.

4.4 Sodium and water homeostasis is mediated mainly by the kidney. The sodium content of the body is maintained by renal excretion and conservation and is intimately linked to the regulation of water content and blood volume. An increase in blood volume increases arterial pressure, renal perfusion and glomerular filtration, which results in an increase in water and sodium excretion. The mechanism maintaining the balance between blood pressure and sodium excretion is known as *pressure natriuresis*.

4.5   Blood pressure regulation is linked to the kidney's ability to excrete or conserve enough sodium to maintain the body's normal sodium content, ECF volume, and blood volume, in response to variations in sodium intake and losses (Folkow, 1982). The physiological processes involved in maintaining blood pressure operate across a continuum entailing many interactive regulatory mechanisms for which the individual and collective physiological thresholds have not been characterised. (A more detailed overview of processes involved in the regulation of the body's sodium content is provided in Annex 6.)

4.6   Changes in the sodium content of the body, either above or below the ideal range, can lead to adverse effects. Changes are brought about by factors that overcome the body's ability to maintain sodium and/or water content. The sodium content increases when the intake exceeds the body's ability to excrete sodium. Deficiency can arise from increased sodium losses (e.g. by chronic diarrhoea) and/or from very low levels of intake.

4.7   There are inevitable losses of sodium from the body, such as through sweating, as well as requirements for the maintenance of ECF volume. The minimal requirement for sodium could therefore be defined as the level of consumption needed to match obligatory losses and maintain function. A restriction in sodium consumption to a level below the requirement induces physiological changes leading to the active retention of sodium in the body, mainly by the kidney.

4.8   Intakes exceeding requirements must be excreted in order to maintain the sodium content of the body. However, there is an upper limit to the rate at which sodium can be lost from the body. Intakes beyond this point cause an increase in sodium content, which in turn causes water to be retained. Short term adjustments may not be manifested; however, if the extent to which the intake exceeds the capacity for excretion is large, or maintained for long periods of time, there are then irreversible changes in the adaptive thresholds which leads ultimately to tissue damage (Folkow, 1982). One important manifestation may be the development of higher blood pressure.

4.9   The capacity of the kidney to regulate the sodium content of the body varies with a number of factors, including age. For example, both the very young and the old have a decreased capacity for salt excretion. Some population groups have a reduced capacity from an earlier age which may be genetic, or a consequence of their habitual dietary consumption during early life. Other dietary and lifestyle factors may exert direct or indirect effects on renal function and thereby alter the renal capacity for sodium excretion.

4.10   The physiological range of sodium required for homeostasis has not been established, i.e. the minimum intake required to match obligatory losses and the upper level beyond which the homeostatic mechanism fails.

4.11   The physiological requirements for sodium were considered throughout life. For adults, the minimal and upper levels of sodium associated with irreversible changes will vary amongst individuals for a variety of reasons, such as age, genetic predisposition, and environmental conditions. Therefore, for the population as a whole, desirable levels of consumption should allow for this variability. (Infants and children are considered in Section 6.)

4.12   Low salt intakes might primarily be expected to have adverse effects on work ability and thermoregulation in high environmental temperatures. In rats, sodium deprivation induced by sodium free diets and diuretic treatment results in impaired thermoregulation (De Garavilla et al, 1990). Severe heat exposure of sodium depleted rats was found to cause problems with food consumption and growth (Francesconi & Hubbard, 1985). In humans, extreme salt depletion, using salt free diets under experimental conditions, causes fatigue, weakness, muscle cramps, as well as psychological effects (McCance, 1935). Extreme depletion, usually caused by medical conditions, can be fatal.

4.13   Estimated requirements for salt intakes of humans exposed to hot environments have ranged between 2-20g per day (0.8-8g/35-347 mmol sodium) (Francesconi et al, 1993). Acute heat stress might be expected to occur when troops, habitually consuming 8-15g salt per day (3.2-6g/139-260 mmol/ sodium), are mobilised from temperate to desert or jungle environments.

4.14   Taylor et al (1944) investigated the relationship of salt intake to heat exhaustion and cardiovascular function in unacclimatised men working in the heat, and the maximum salt intake required in these conditions. They found that for unacclimatised men working for 2-3.5 days in the heat (49°C), sweating 5-8 litres per day, the maximum salt requirement was not more than 15-17g (6-6.8g/261-296 mmol sodium). No physiological advantage was gained by increasing levels of salt to 30g (12g/522 mmol sodium) per day. Those consuming 4-8g salt (1.6-3.2g/70-139 mmol sodium) daily did not drink sufficient water and were more likely to suffer acute heat exhaustion caused by impaired cardiovascular function.

4.15   A heat acclimatisation study (Francesconi et al, 1993) compared responses of military personnel exposed to heat (41°C), over 10 days, on diets which contained either 8g of salt (3.2g/139 mmol sodium) or 4g salt (1.6g/70 mmol sodium) per day and where dehydration was avoided. The endocrine responses demonstrated adaptation to both levels of salt intake. Within 10 days of heat exposure, there were significant reductions in exercise-induced heart rate, rectal temperature, urinary sodium, and perceived exertion. There were no significant differences in these variables between the two groups. This study suggests that healthy individuals can adapt to lower salt intakes at high temperatures.

4.16   Lowest average intakes of sodium consistent with apparent good health, in individuals or populations, have ranged between 69-920mg/3-40 mmol per day (1.75-2.3g salt) (DH, 1991) and populations surviving on as little as 5mg/0.2 mmol sodium per day (0.01g salt) have been reported (Intersalt Cooperative Research Group, 1988).

4.17   The suggestion of an inverse relationship between salt consumption and cardiovascular outcomes (Alderman et al, 1995; Alderman et al, 1998) is considered in a later section of the report (see paragraphs 4.68 & 4.70).

Summary and conclusions

4.18   There is little evidence that, in a temperate climate such as that of the UK, salt intakes of 4-6g per day (70-100 mmol/1.6-2.4g sodium) would have any adverse physiological effects on a healthy population.

4.19   No basis was found for a revision of the Dietary Reference Values for sodium or a change to the 1994 COMA recommendation for a target salt intake of 6g/day (2.4g/100 mmol sodium) for the adult population. The target of 6g/day is higher than the RNI for sodium (1.6g or 70 mmol sodium/4g salt) and substantially greater than the salt intake required to maintain the sodium content of the body. A salt intake of 6g/day remains an achievable population target and not an optimal or ideal level.

Salt sensitivity

4.20   The heterogeneous response to the effect of salt on blood pressure has given rise to the concept of *salt sensitive* and *salt resistant* individuals within populations. It is based on the idea that some individuals might be more susceptible than others to salt-induced effects on blood pressure and has been used as an argument against public health measures for salt reduction, in favour of an individual clinical approach.

4.21 Salt sensitivity has been defined as a change in blood pressure in response to sodium loading or depletion although there has been no consistency between studies in the sodium load administered or in the nature of the response elicited. (See Annex 7 for the different criteria and methods that have been applied to assess salt sensitivity.)

4.22 Studies to test the reproducibility of the effect of sodium loading and depletion on blood pressure have yielded conflicting results. Three studies that examined individuals at different times showed reasonable reproducibility (Overlack et al, 1993; Sharma et al, 1989; Weinberger & Finberg, 1991) whilst in other studies, reproducibility was found to be poor (Gerdts et al, 1999; Mattes & Falkner, 1999; Zoccali et al, 1996).

4.23 It has been suggested that salt sensitivity might be a transient phenomenon during the pathogenesis and development of hypertension and occurs as a result of subtle acquired renal injury (Johnson et al, 2002). Subtle renal injury impairs sodium excretion and the ensuing sodium retention leads to an increase in blood pressure.

4.24 The phenomenon of *reverse* salt sensitivity has also been reported (Ruppert et al, 1993). Acute extreme salt restriction (1.2g salt/0.48g or 20 mmol sodium) of 163 subjects was associated with an increase in mean arterial blood pressure greater than or equal to 5 mm Hg in 15% of the participants. This effect has not been reported for more moderate intakes of salt.

Prevalence of salt sensitivity

4.25   Due to lack of uniformity in study criteria and techniques and because most studies have involved small numbers of subjects, estimates of the prevalence of salt sensitivity have been wide-ranging. Variability in the populations studied, particularly the age of subjects, ethnic origin, obesity, and level of intake of other dietary minerals, are also likely to have affected prevalence estimates.

4.26   Taking all these factors into account, a higher frequency of salt sensitivity has been observed in adults with hypertension. Estimates of prevalence have ranged from 29-60% in hypertensive populations and 15-46% in normotensive populations, although the larger studies have indicated that over 50% of a hypertensive population and approximately 25% of a normotensive population are salt sensitive (Weinberger et al, 1986; Sullivan, 1991).

4.27   Salt sensitivity has been more frequently observed among black rather than white subjects in both normotensive and hypertensive populations and in older rather than younger subjects. However change in prevalence with age has received limited investigation and salt sensitivity has been observed in African American adolescents (Wilson et al, 1999).

Salt sensitivity as an independent predictor of cardiovascular events

4.28   Morimoto et al (1997) examined the relationship between salt sensitivity and occurrence of cardiovascular events in 156 Japanese hypertensive patients without other pre-existing disorders. Patients were followed up for a mean of

7.3 years and cardiovascular events were found to be twice as common in the patients previously classified as salt sensitive[10]. Significantly more patients in the salt sensitive group had left ventricular hypertrophy. Salt sensitivity as a cardiovascular risk factor was found to be independent of other risk factors such as smoking and blood pressure.

4.29   A study by Weinberger et al (2001) obtained long-term follow-up data for 596 subjects (85% of an original cohort) who had been assessed for salt sensitivity[11] 27 years previously. The cohort included men, women, African-Americans, and a diverse age range (18-80y at baseline). In normotensive subjects aged over 25 years, who were identified as salt sensitive when initially studied, there was an increased risk of cardiovascular events and death which was similar to that of hypertensive subjects. The investigators had not controlled for smoking as a cardiovascular risk factor.

Summary and conclusions

4.30   There is no agreed definition or clinical criteria to identify salt sensitivity. Sodium loading and depletion protocols have involved extreme manipulations, which are unrealistic representations of variations in dietary salt intakes within actual populations and may not reflect long-term blood pressure responses to salt intakes on a population basis.

---

10 Salt sensitivity was defined as a 10% or greater difference in mean arterial blood pressure between a low salt diet (1-3g salt/0.4-1.2g or 17.4-52 mmol sodium per day for one week) and a high salt diet (12-15g salt/4.8-6g or 209-261 mmol sodium per day for one week).
11 Participants with a change in mean arterial blood pressure of at least 10 mm Hg in response to intravenous saline administration and rapid diuretic-induced sodium and volume depletion, had been classified as salt sensitive.

4.31   It is clear that there is a spectrum of responses to dietary salt exposure and all individuals will display an inability to cope with excess intakes at a certain level. It is possible that some individuals will display elevated blood pressure at lower levels of salt intake than others. Since the phenomenon of salt sensitivity has not been characterised it is not yet possible to identify and develop predictive markers, including genetic polymorphisms, for individuals or populations with this propensity. The greatest benefits are likely to be achieved by taking a population approach to reducing salt intake.

Evidence for an association between salt intake and blood pressure

Animal studies

4.32   Most animal studies on the effects of increased salt intake on blood pressure have primarily involved rodent models. However, routine veterinary data of chimpanzees in a research institute fed on a diet of monkey chow (containing 6-12g salt or 2.4-4.8g/100-200 mmol sodium per day) supplemented with fruit, revealed age-related changes in blood pressure analogous to those observed in urbanised human populations (Eichberg and Shade, 1987). Based on these observations, Denton et al (1995) examined the effect of increased levels of salt on the blood pressure of a colony of 26 chimpanzees (aged 5-18y) maintained on a vegetable and fruit diet.

4.33   The chimpanzees were randomised into two groups of 13 animals. The control group was fed the usual diet which was low in sodium and high in potassium. The intervention group was fed increasing amounts of salt over 89 weeks: 5g/d (2g/87 mmol sodium) for 19 weeks, 10g/d (4g/174 mmol sodium) for 3 weeks, and 15g/d (6g/261 mmol sodium) for 67 weeks. Salt intake was assessed from 24-hour urine collections by means of catheterisation. They were then returned to their usual diet and blood pressure continued to be monitored for the following 6 months.

4.34   Compared with controls, after 19 weeks on 5g/d salt (2g/87 mmol sodium) mean systolic pressure increased by 12 mm Hg; increasing salt intake resulted in further increases up to 33 mm Hg on 15g salt (6g/261 mmol sodium) per day. There were clear differences in sodium excretion between intervention and controls. Blood pressures returned to normal on withdrawal of the intervention. During the salt intervention the weights of the animals increased significantly compared to controls.

4.35   These results show that increased salt intake in chimpanzees causes a large rise in blood pressure and demonstrate the dose-responsive nature of the relationship. Additionally, in the intervention group, 70% of the chimpanzees responded with a notable rise in blood pressure and 30% showed a small or no change, illustrating the variability of the response to salt intakes. In this study, salt was the only variable that was changed; all other variables, such as potassium intake and social conditions, remained constant. The high potassium intakes, characteristic of a fruit and vegetable diet, did not prevent the increased blood pressure responses observed in the intervention group.

Human epidemiological studies

- Cross-sectional studies

4.36   A number of migration studies of population groups moving from rural areas with low salt intakes to urban environments of high salt intake have reported increases in blood pressure similar to that of the host population (He et al, 1991; Poulter et al, 1990). Such data are difficult to interpret and are inconclusive, in terms of the effect of salt consumption, because of the number of confounding factors associated with lifestyle and environmental changes.

4.37   The International Study of Salt & Blood Pressure (Intersalt Co-operative Research Group, 1988) collected data on 24-hour urinary sodium excretion and blood pressure of over 10,000 adults in 52 population samples from 32 countries. Significant positive associations were found between sodium excretion and both systolic and diastolic blood pressures. When four centres with unacculturated populations that had very low salt intakes were removed from the analysis, the overall association between sodium intakes and blood pressure was not statistically significant; however, an association was found between salt intake and increase in blood pressure with age. Body mass index (BMI) and alcohol had independent effects on blood pressure. As the age-blood pressure relationship was not part of the original hypothesis for the study, there has been a difference of opinion about the weight that might be placed on these observations.

4.38   Subsequent re-analysis of the data, which adjusted for regression dilution caused by measurement errors incurred in the study (Elliott et al, 1993; Elliott et al, 1996), found stronger associations. There have been suggestions that the correction factors used may have been overestimated (Day, 1997; Davey Smith & Phillips, 1997).

4.39   The International Co-operation Study of Macronutrients and Blood Pressure (INTERMAP), with data from a total of 4,680 participants in 17 populations from the UK, US, China and Japan, is still in progress (Elliott; personal communication, 2002).

- Intervention studies

4.40   In reviewing studies on the relationship between salt and blood pressure with morbidity/mortality outcomes, consideration was given to the design of the studies, particularly the method used to measure dietary exposure to salt (see paragraph 1.7) and allowance for the main cardiovascular risk factors.

4.41   Greater weight was placed on studies of four or more weeks in duration as adaptive responses to changes in dietary salt intakes may take more than a few days to become apparent.

4.42   When reviewing intervention studies, a distinction was made between trials of efficacy relating to dietary manipulations and trials of effectiveness utilising dietary advice. The intervention studies reviewed are included in Annex 8.

    − Dietary manipulation

4.43   The Dietary Approaches to Stop Hypertension (DASH) trial (Appel et al, 1997) assessed the effects of dietary patterns on blood pressure. A group of 459 normotensive and hypertensive adults (22y or older) received a control diet (low in fruit, vegetables and dairy products, with a fat content typical of the average US diet) for three weeks. Participants were then randomised to receive one of three diets for eight weeks: the control diet, a diet rich in fruit and vegetables, or a combination diet (the DASH diet), rich in fruit, vegetables, low-fat dairy products, and with reduced saturated and total fat. The salt content of each diet was similar. Weight, physical activity, and alcohol were held constant for all the groups.

4.44 The results demonstrated that compared to a typical US diet, a diet rich in fruits, vegetables, and low-fat dairy products (the DASH diet), significantly reduced mean blood pressure by 5.5/3.0 mm Hg. The diet rich in fruit and vegetables produced a significant reduction of 2.8 mm Hg in systolic blood pressure but not in diastolic blood pressure (which was reduced by 1.1 mm Hg). Among subjects with hypertension, the DASH diet significantly reduced blood pressure by 11.4/5.5 mm Hg and in those without hypertension by 3.5/2.1 mm Hg. The effects appeared within 2 weeks of participants being placed on the DASH diet and persisted for the remaining six weeks of the intervention.

4.45 The follow-up DASH Sodium trial (Sacks et al, 2001a) examined the combined effect of the DASH diet and reduced salt intake. 412 participants (aged 37-59y) were randomly assigned to the control or DASH diet for a period of three months. Each subject consumed their allocated diet for 30 consecutive days at each of three levels of salt: high (9g salt/3.6g or 150 mmol sodium), intermediate (6g salt/2.4g or 100 mmol sodium); and low (3g salt/1.2g or 50 mmol sodium). The potassium intakes were greater on the DASH diet than in the controls, but were kept the same for all levels of salt intake (approximately 1.6g potassium on control diet and 3g on DASH diet). Weight remained stable in all groups.

4.46   Reducing salt intake from the higher to the lower level significantly reduced blood pressure by 6.7/3.5 mm Hg on the control diet and by 3.0/1.6 mm Hg on the DASH diet. The combined effects on blood pressure of the DASH diet and low salt intake were greater than either of the interventions alone and were 8.9/4.5 mm Hg below the control diet at the high salt level. With this combination, mean systolic blood pressure was 11.5 mm Hg lower in participants with hypertension, and 7.1 mm Hg lower in participants without hypertension.

4.47   Results of the DASH Sodium trial showed that blood pressure was reduced in a stepwise fashion in response to a reduction in the salt intake on both the DASH diet and the control diet. The effects were observed in those with and without hypertension, in both sexes, and across racial groups.

4.48   One criticism of the DASH Sodium trial was that it concentrated on the favourable effect of lowering salt on blood pressure to the exclusion of other harmful physiological effects, for example, an increase in the plasma levels of renin (Alderman 2001). McCarron (2001) claimed that adequate mineral intake from the DASH diet was far more important than salt in determining blood pressure and argued that from a clinically applicable view, any effect of salt restriction on blood pressure was limited to hypertensive black females in the study population. Another assertion was that only data for effects on systolic blood pressure of the different groups (i.e. defined by ethnic background, sex, presence or absence of hypertension) were presented (Petitti and Freedman, 2001) and that diastolic blood pressure might be more important in relation to the risk of stroke and cardiovascular disease.

4.49   In response to these criticisms, the authors (Sacks et al, 2001b) argued that diuretic therapy, which prevents cardiovascular disease, also raises plasma renin. Additionally, in a large sample of the general population, plasma renin level was not associated with cardiovascular disease (Meade et al, 1993). The authors accepted that susceptibility to salt may vary in the population, however the effects of salt reduction in the DASH Sodium trial were qualitatively similar among all subgroups but quantitatively different. Systolic blood pressure was prespecified as the trial's primary outcome because it has been more closely linked than diastolic blood pressure to cardiovascular disease (Weinberger et al, 1986).

4.50   The Prospective Studies Collaboration (2002) found systolic blood pressure to be a more informative measure of risk than diastolic blood pressure, irrespective of age. *British Hypertension Society Guidelines* (Ramsay et al, 1999) assign equal importance to systolic and diastolic blood pressure in relation to cardiovascular disease risks (Stamler et al, 1993). Outcome trials of antihypertensive treatment based on thresholds of diastolic or systolic hypertension have shown similar reductions in cardiovascular disease events (Gueyffier et al, 1997).

- Dietary advice

4.51   The Trials of Hypertension Prevention (TOHP) Phase II (TOHP Collaborative Research Group, 1997) was a longitudinal study that evaluated the effects of reduced salt intake (target of 4.8g salt/1.8g or 80 mmol sodium) and weight loss, either alone or in combination, on blood pressure. Participants in the study were moderately overweight with high normal blood pressures and thus representative of the majority of industrialised populations rather than extremes.

4.52   At 6 months, sodium excretion was reduced by 78 mmol (1.8g sodium/4.6g salt) in the salt reduction group and by 64 mmol (1.5g sodium/3.7g salt) in the combined intervention group, achieving salt intake levels of 6.1g (2.4g/104 mmol sodium) and 7.3g (2.9g/124 mmol sodium) respectively. Compared to the usual care group, systolic and diastolic blood pressures were significantly lowered by 2.9/1.6 mm Hg in the salt reduction group, by 3.7/2.7 mm Hg in the weight loss group, and by 4.0/2.8 mm Hg in the combined intervention group.

4.53   Effects were reduced at 36 months. Diastolic blood pressure reductions remained significant only in the weight loss group and systolic blood pressure reductions were small but significant for the salt reduction group (1.2 mm Hg) and the weight loss group (1.3 mm Hg). Sodium excretion increased significantly over time and at 36 months, there were only small but significant differences from the usual care group of 40 mmol/d (0.9g sodium/2.3g salt) for the salt reduction group and 24 mmol/d (0.6g sodium/1.4g salt) for the combined group.

4.54   The greater magnitude of the short-term compared to long-term effects reflects the difficulties individuals face in making substantial changes to their diet and complying with dietary restrictions, particularly in relation to reduced salt intake.

4.55   The Trial of Nonpharmacologic Interventions in the Elderly (TONE) (Whelton et al, 1998) evaluated the effects of salt reduction (target of 4.8g salt/1.8g or 80 mmol sodium) and weight loss, alone and combined, in older hypertensives (aged 60-80y) whose blood pressures were controlled with one antihypertensive drug. Weight loss and salt reduction in the diet were achievable and, where both interventions were successful, more individuals were able to stop and remain off medication. The greater success of the salt reduction and weight loss intervention in this age group may reflect an increased motivation to reduce dependence on antihypertensive medication.

   – Meta-analyses of intervention trials

4.56   Several meta-analyses (summarised in Annex 9) have been conducted to pool the results of randomised controlled intervention trials investigating the effect of salt reduction on hypertension (Midgley et al, 1996; Cutler et al, 1997; Ebrahim & Davey Smith 1998; Graudal et al, 1998; Alam & Johnson 1999). Three suggest that decreases in blood pressure in response to sodium reduction are not sufficient to justify population-wide advice to lower salt intakes (Midgley et al, 1996; Ebrahim & Davey Smith, 1998; Graudal et al, 1998). Criticism of these meta-analyses have centred on the inclusion of trials of short duration, and trials that compared the effects of acute salt loading followed by severe depletion which does not reflect the actual situation with habitual diets.

4.57 A meta-analysis by MacGregor and He (2002) only included studies with modest salt reductions and a duration of at least four weeks. The DASH Sodium trial, which had not been published at the time of previous meta-analyses, was also included. Seventeen trials in hypertensives and 11 trials in normotensives were combined and pooled estimates found significant reductions in blood pressure of 4.96/2.73 mm Hg in hypertensives and 2.03/0.97 mm Hg in normotensives. These results demonstrate that, on a population-wide basis, a modest reduction in salt intake for a period of four or more weeks has a significant effect on blood pressure in hypertensive and normotensive individuals.

4.58 A systematic review by Hooper et al (2002) assessed the long-term effects of advice to reduce dietary salt in adults with and without hypertension. Eleven trials were included with follow-up from 6 months to 7 years. Pooled estimates at 6-12 months showed significant reductions of 2.5/1.2 mm Hg in systolic and diastolic blood pressures. At 13-60 months after initial advice, a significant reduction (1.1 mm Hg) only remained for systolic blood pressure. 24-hour sodium excretion was reduced by 48 mmol/d (1.1g sodium/2.8g salt) at 6-12 months and by 35.5 mmol/d (0.8g sodium/2.1g) at 13-60 months. There was significant heterogeneity in sodium excretion measurements, which could not be explained by trial quality.

Summary and conclusions

4.59 The evidence of an association between dietary salt intakes and blood pressure has increased since 1994. The data have been consistent in various study populations, including different ethnic groups, and across the age range in adults.

4.60   The DASH Sodium trial and the study on chimpanzees clearly demonstrate dose-responsive effects of salt on blood pressure. In the DASH Sodium trial, the greatest reductions in blood pressure were observed when the DASH diet, rich in fruits, vegetables and low-fat dairy products and reduced saturated and total fat, was combined with a low salt diet. The clear and distinct effect of salt on blood pressure indicates that lowering salt intakes as part of a healthy whole diet strategy would be most effective as a population-based approach to lowering blood pressures.

4.61   The systematic review on long-term effects of advice to reduce dietary salt levels (Hooper et al, 2002), showed that the significant blood pressure reductions observed at 6-12 months, were not sustained over time. As most dietary salt intake originates from processed food, this illustrates the difficulties faced by individuals in maintaining a low salt diet and supports the view that a targeted individual approach to salt reduction is inappropriate. A population-based approach is required to achieve a sustained reduction in salt intake. With the continued co-operation of the food industry to lower salt levels in processed foods, a gradual lowering of population salt intakes could be achieved over time.

4.62   A reduction in the dietary salt intake of the population would lower the blood pressure risk for the whole population.

Morbidity and premature mortality

4.63   Although clear effects of salt on blood pressure have been observed, the long-term effects on health and premature mortality outcomes are less certain.

Animal studies

4.64   Experimental evidence from rats has shown that high salt diets (containing 8% salt) may accelerate death from cerebral arterial disease even in the absence of rises in blood pressure in comparison with rats on lower salt (0.3%) diets over a 15 week experimental period (Tobian & Hanlon, 1990).

Human studies

4.65   The design of the studies that were considered, assessing effects of either salt intake or blood pressure levels on morbidity and premature mortality outcomes, can be found in Annex 8. The design issues outlined in Section 1 and allowances for the main cardiovascular risk factors, were taken into account.

- Cardiovascular disease

    - Cross-sectional studies

4.66   Analysis of sodium excretion data from the 12 Western European countries which participated in the Intersalt Study showed a relationship with stroke mortality in univariate analysis, which remained significant when adjusted for BMI (Perry & Beevers, 1992). However, sodium excretion and alcohol intake were highly inter-correlated and it was not possible to demonstrate an effect independent of alcohol intake. Stroke mortality was not related to systolic blood pressure in this analysis.

4.67   The WHO Cardiovascular Diseases and Alimentary Comparison (CARDIAC) Study (Yamori et al, 1994), included 55 centres in 24 countries and examined 100 men and 100 women (aged 48-56y) randomly selected from the population. Blood pressure was measured in a standardised manner and estimates of sodium intake were determined from 24-hour urine collections. Age-adjusted stroke mortality was reported to be significantly and positively associated with urinary sodium excretion in men and to the sodium/potassium ratio in both sexes.

–   Prospective studies

4.68   An analysis of data from the National Health and Nutritional Examination Survey I (NHANES I) reported an inverse association between dietary sodium intake and all-cause and cardiovascular disease mortality (Alderman et al, 1998). The authors acknowledged the limitations of the analysis, including the reliability of the measures based on a single 24-hour dietary recall, for both sodium and energy intakes. The estimated sodium intakes in NHANES also did not include salt used in cooking or at the table. Hypertensive persons, who may have been advised to reduce their salt intake, were included in the analysis and there was no control for smoking as a confounder.

4.69   An alternative analysis of the NHANES I data (He et al, 1999) which controlled for smoking status, found that in participants who were overweight, sodium intake was associated with increased frequency of stroke, mortality from coronary heart disease, cardiovascular disease, and all causes.

4.70   An earlier claim, that a reduction in salt intake increases the risk of myocardial infarction (Alderman et al, 1995), was based on an observational study of a group of 2937 patients with drug treated hypertension followed up for a median of 3.5 years. 24-hour urinary excretion of sodium was inversely related to the incidence of myocardial infarction. However, the baseline sodium excretion was only measured once, after patients had been advised to avoid high salt foods for 4-5 days before the 24-hour urine collection. This measurement was therefore not an accurate reflection of habitual intake and, in some cases, the 24-hour urine collections may have been incomplete. The basis of this study was not in fact concerned with salt ingestion and the salt restriction phase was carried out to allow classification of the subjects according to renin profiles.

4.71   Tunstall-Pedoe et al (1997) analysed data from a large prospective cohort in the Scottish Heart Health Study. 72% of the original cohort of 11629 men and women were followed up for an average of 7.6 years, and initial results were from univariate analysis only. 24-hour urinary sodium excretion did not predict coronary heart disease in men. In women, the gradient was borderline positive for all coronary heart disease. Increased potassium excretion was associated with significant protection against all coronary heart disease in men.

4.72   A prospective study in Finland (Tuomilehto et al, 2001) followed 1173 men and 1263 women (aged 25-64y) over 10 years, for whom complete 24-hour urine sodium excretion and cardiovascular endpoint data were available. The risk of death from coronary heart disease and cardiovascular disease, and incidence of coronary heart disease but not stroke, rose significantly with increasing sodium excretion. A stepwise increase (hazard ratio of 1.5) was observed for each 100 mmol/2.4g (6g salt) increase in sodium excretion. Data were adjusted for sex and for cardiovascular disease risk factors such as smoking, body mass index, and serum cholesterol.

4.73 Mortality and cardiovascular outcomes were examined in a systematic review on the long-term effects of advice to reduce dietary salt in adults (Hooper et al, 2002). The 11 trials included in the review provided few data on mortality and cardiovascular events and such data were inconsistently reported.

• Other outcomes

– Left ventricular hypertrophy

4.74 Left ventricular hypertrophy (LVH) is a powerful risk factor for cardiovascular disease (Levy et al, 1989). In the Treatment of Mild Hypertension Study (TOMHS), dietary salt intake, assessed by sodium excretion over 24-hours, was found to be an important determinant of left ventricular mass (LVM) (Beil & Schmieder, 1995).

4.75 TOMHS, a randomised double-blind clinical trial of 844 mild hypertensives, compared five classes of antihypertensive drugs and placebo in conjunction with nutritional advice given for weight loss, reducing sodium and alcohol intake and increasing physical activity (Liebson et al, 1995). The outcome measure of interest was echocardiographically measured LVM as a risk factor for cardiovascular disease events. Follow-up was over 48 months and results showed that nutritional advice alone, specifically weight reduction and limitation of salt intake, was as effective in reducing LVM as combined nutritional and drug therapy, despite greater blood pressure reductions with additional drug therapy.

– Bone health

4.76   High salt intakes have been associated with increases in urinary calcium loss and it has been hypothesised that this may contribute to osteoporosis. It has been estimated that urinary calcium levels increase by approximately 1 mmol per 100 mmol sodium intake (Nordin et al, 1993).

4.77   Reports on the effects of salt on bone biomarkers have been inconsistent. Most of the studies in this area have involved small numbers of subjects and the interventions have been of very short duration.

4.78   McParland et al (1989) found that a salt intake of 10.2g/d (3.9g/170 mmol sodium) for 7 days caused a significant increase in biomarkers of bone resorption in 10 postmenopausal women. Evans et al (1997) investigated the effects of 18g salt (6.9g/300 mmol sodium) per day on 11 premenopausal and 11 post menopausal women over 7 days. On the high salt diet, there was a significant increase in a marker of bone resorption in postmenopausal women, which was not observed in premenopausal women.

4.79   Other studies have shown no effect of high intakes of salt. In an 8-day study of 14 postmenopausal women (Lietz et al, 1997), no effects on bone resorption markers were observed at levels of 10.2g/d of salt (3.9g/170 mmol sodium). Ginty et al (1998) found no effects of 10.8g salt/d (4.1g/180 mmol sodium) for 14 days on markers of bone turnover in 29 women.

4.80   A larger study of 60 postmenopausal women (Sellmeyer et al, 2002) found that an increase in dietary salt to 13.5g/d (5.2g/225 mmol sodium) for 4 weeks, was associated with a significant increase in excretion of bone resorption markers. This effect was prevented by oral administration of potassium citrate suggesting that at high salt intakes, increased consumption of fruit and vegetables, which are rich in potassium, may be beneficial in the prevention of bone loss.

4.81   In an ancillary study of the DASH Sodium trial, bone turnover was investigated in 187 participants aged 23-76y (Lin et al, 2000). No effects were observed in markers of bone formation and resorption at the three levels of salt intake. The DASH diet itself, consumed for 30 days, reduced bone turnover at all levels of salt intake regardless of age, race, gender, and hypertension status.

Summary and conclusions

4.82   Although studies which have collected 24-hour urine prospectively suggest that a high salt intake has adverse effects on cardiovascular disease mortality, there are insufficient reliable data on morbidity and premature mortality outcomes to reach clear conclusions. The available evidence reflects the inherent difficulties of undertaking large scale studies of long duration that are required to assess long-term outcomes and the problems of isolating the effects of salt intake from other factors.

4.83   The studies on LVH suggest that high salt intakes cause increases in left ventricular mass independently of blood pressure.

4.84   There are insufficient data to assess effects of high salt intake on bone health and further research is required in this area.

5 The Role of Other Factors in the Development of Hypertension

5.1 The development of hypertension is dependent on the interaction of dietary factors, alcohol consumption, obesity and its association with metabolic syndrome, lack of activity, and genetic predisposition. These factors were not within the remit of this review and are only considered briefly.

Other dietary factors

5.2 Potassium, calcium, and magnesium have specifically been credited with having significant effects on blood pressure. Other micronutrients may also be involved but the mechanisms remain unclear. It is difficult to relate blood pressure levels to specific nutrients because of strong correlations between dietary intakes of potassium, magnesium, calcium, and fibre.

5.3 The evidence regarding the benefits of increased intake of fruit and vegetables on blood pressure is consistent. Margetts et al (1986) found that switching to a vegetarian diet reduced systolic blood pressure by 5 mm Hg over a 6-week period. The DASH trial (Appel et al, 1997), which assessed the effects of dietary patterns on blood pressure, confirmed the importance of multiple factors in the diet for blood pressure control.

5.4   A randomised controlled trial by John et al (2002) used dietary advice to encourage an increase in consumption of fruit and vegetables to at least five portions a day, for a 6-month period. Compared to the control group, blood pressure in the intervention group decreased significantly by 4.0/1.5 mm Hg.

Alcohol

5.5   Alcohol intake is an independent risk factor associated with hypertension (Marmot et al, 1994). A meta-analysis of 15 randomised controlled trials, with 2234 participants, assessed the effects of alcohol reduction on blood pressure (Xin et al, 2001). The mean baseline alcohol consumption of participants was 3-6 drinks per day (units of alcohol were not stated). An average 67% reduction in consumption of alcohol was associated with a significant lowering of mean systolic and diastolic blood pressures by 3.31/2.04 mm Hg and a dose-response relationship was observed.

Body weight

5.6   Blood pressure rises with increasing adiposity (Chen et al, 1995) and weight reduction in hypertensive patients is associated with a decline in blood pressure (Mulrow et al, 2002). There is a tendency for a number of cardiovascular risk factors, including hypertension, to occur together. This clustering of risk factors has been termed metabolic syndrome or Syndrome X and encompasses hypertension, obesity, glucose intolerance, insulin resistance, dyslipaedemia, and lack of activity. As all these factors mutually reinforce each other, an improvement in any one of them will impact on the others.

Physical activity

5.7 Increased physical activity has been associated with reductions in systolic and diastolic blood pressure in hypertensive and normotensive individuals although the reductions have been shown to be greater for hypertensives (Lesniak and Dubbert 2001). A meta-analysis, of 54 randomised controlled trials involving 2419 participants, on the effect of aerobic exercise on blood pressure (Whelton et al, 2002) found that aerobic exercise was associated with a significant reduction in mean systolic and diastolic blood pressure (3.84/2.58 mm Hg). Aerobic exercise was associated with a reduction in blood pressure in both hypertensives and normotensives as well as in overweight and normal weight individuals.

Genetic predisposition

5.8 Studies have shown that polymorphisms in certain genes, such as the angiotensinogen gene, might be implicated in the blood pressure response to a high salt intake (Hunt et al 1998; Svetkey et al 2001). Multiple genetic loci may be involved in blood pressure regulation and any single polymorphism by itself may have a relatively small impact on blood pressure level. Little is known about the interactions between genetic polymorphisms and dietary factors in the regulation of blood pressure and current studies have limited statistical power to examine such interactions (Corvol et al, 1999).

Summary and conclusions

5.9 High salt intake is one of a number of risk factors, including obesity and alcohol consumption, that increase the risk of developing hypertension. A generally healthy diet that is rich in fruit and vegetables has been shown to be protective.

5.10 Public health strategies to reduce blood pressure levels should be based on a general healthy lifestyle approach and include strategies for increasing physical activity and reducing alcohol consumption and levels of obesity in the UK.

5.11 It is probable that future research will identify multiple genetic polymorphisms that contribute to the individual risk of high blood pressure and varied responses to salt.

6 Infants and Children

Physiological requirements for sodium

6.1   In the first 6 months of life, the level of sodium in breast milk is adequate to support normal growth and development and, compared to adults, the ability to excrete sodium loads is reduced (Spitzer et al, 1982). Mean sodium concentrations of breast milk have been reported to range from 7 mmol/L (160mg sodium/0.4g salt) in early lactation to 5 mmol/L (120mg sodium/0.3g salt) or less in later lactation (Fomon, 1993). The sodium content of infant formulas are prescribed by the *Infant Formula and Follow-on Formula Regulations* (1995). The requirements for premature infants were not considered.

6.2   For children aged over 6 months no data could be found on the range of intakes required for normal sodium homeostasis. The Dietary Reference Values agreed by COMA for ages 7 months upwards were calculated factorially (DH, 1991) and were considered appropriate.

6.3   The target salt intakes for infants and children have been estimated on the same basis used to derive the recommended target salt intake for adults, i.e. an increase in the RNI by a factor of 1.5, and have been rounded to the nearest whole number (Table 2). The age bands are based on dietary patterns at different stages of growth. Relative to salt and energy intake recommendations, these targets are proportionate to those for adults.

Table 2: Reference nutrient intakes (RNI) for sodium & target
average salt intakes for infants & children

Age	RNI		Target average salt intake (g/d)
	sodium mmol/d (mg/d)	salt (g/d)	
0-6 months*	10.5 (242)	0.60	‹ 1
7-12 months*	14.5 (334)	0.84	1
1-3 years	22 (500)	1.28	2
4-6 years	30 (700)	1.80	3
7-10 years	50 (1200)	3.06	5
11-14 years	70 (1600)	4.08	6

* The RNI for infants aged 0-6m represent the average RNI of the 0-3m &
3-6m age groups; the RNI for infants aged 7-12m represents the average
RNI of the 7-9m & 10-12m age groups.)

6.4   The average salt intake target recommended for each age
group does not represent an optimal or ideal consumption level
for infants and children but an achievable population goal.

Blood pressure

6.5   Blood pressure of children is lower than that of adults.
Population level data on reference blood pressure ranges of
children are not available although values have been
published from a cross-sectional study of school children in
Newcastle (O'Sullivan et al, 1999). There are also no defined
clinical blood pressure thresholds for the diagnosis of
hypertension in children (Blood Pressure Association;
personal communication, 2002).

6.6   Robust studies examining the effect of salt intake on blood pressure in children are lacking. The studies that have taken place are difficult to interpret because of methodological constraints (Simons-Morton & Obarzanek, 1997). Therefore, the approach used to assess the evidence for adults could not be applied.

6.7   Sinaiko et al (1993) examined the effects of decreasing the dietary sodium/potassium ratio on blood pressure during adolescence. A group of 210 adolescents (aged 13y at baseline), in the upper 15% of the blood pressure distribution of 19452 children, were assigned to either a low sodium diet, potassium supplementation, or placebo. Blood pressure was measured every three months and 24-hour urine collections were obtained yearly. At baseline, the mean salt intake for girls was 7.8g/d (3.1g/133 mmol sodium) and for boys was 8.3g/d (3.3g/142 mmol sodium). None of the subjects were able to achieve the target intake of 4g of salt per day (1.6g/70 mmol sodium). Only the girls showed a significant decrease in 24-hour urinary sodium excretion, achieving the greatest reduction at 24 months with a salt intake of 6g/d (2.4g/100 mmol sodium). For boys, significant yearly increases in blood pressure were observed with no differences between the three groups. For girls, the yearly rate of rise in blood pressure for the low sodium and potassium supplementation groups were substantially lower than for the placebo group, although this was only significant for the low sodium group.

6.8   A longitudinal study in the Netherlands followed 233 children (aged 5-17y) over an average period of seven years (Geleijnse et al, 1990). Analysis of annual blood pressure measurements found no significant association between sodium excretion and change in blood pressure over time. There was a significant inverse association between the change in mean systolic blood pressure over time and potassium intake. A significant association was also observed between the sodium to potassium ratio and increases in systolic blood pressure over time.

6.9 Evidence from a cross-sectional study of 134 children (aged 8-17y) suggests that small increases in blood pressure can have a detrimental effect on health (Aristimuno et al, 1984). Following a series of blood pressure measurements of 1604 children, over a 4-month period, 90 children with blood pressure in the upper 10% and 44 children with blood pressure in the middle range (50-60th percentile) of the group were selected to evaluate differences in left ventricular voltages between these two blood pressure levels. Subtle electrocardiographic changes were detected in those with blood pressure levels in the upper 10% of the group and some showed signs of left ventricular hypertrophy (LVH) which could not be fully explained by measurement of other anthropometric variables. This finding is notable as LVH is a strong risk factor for cardiovascular disease in adults.

Body weight

6.10 Lurbe et al (2000) described the relationship between sodium excretion and ambulatory blood pressure values in 3-19 year olds. Body weight and sodium excretion were directly associated with systolic blood pressure, however this relationship was modified in obese children who had higher systolic blood pressures than the non-obese at the same sodium excretion levels. It is possible that there is a level of renal dysfunction in obesity which impairs sodium reabsorption and resets pressure natriuresis. However, in those children with highest sodium excretion, differences in blood pressure between obese and non-obese were smaller, and the investigators suggested that there may be a subset of children and adolescents with reduced capacity to excrete sodium, in whom blood pressure is raised.

6.11   Although heavier children have higher blood pressures than less heavy children at the same age, having first degree relatives with high blood pressure also increases the likelihood of higher blood pressure in children (St. George et al, 1990). A similar relationship is found for obesity (Power & Parsons, 2000).

6.12   The rising trend of obesity in children and adolescents is increasingly becoming a cause for concern (Chinn & Rona, 2001) and reinforces the need to tackle all factors, including salt intakes, which potentially contribute toward rises in blood pressure levels.

Early life experience

6.13   Some evidence has suggested that exposure to increased dietary sodium in early life may *programme* the development of higher blood pressure later in life.

6.14   A follow-up study of 545 children (81% of an original cohort), for whom detailed infant feeding histories had been collected in the first two years of life, found that breastfeeding in infancy was associated with lower blood pressure in later childhood (average age 7.3y) (Wilson et al, 1998). Systolic blood pressure was significantly higher in children who had been exclusively fed non-human milk (94.2 mm Hg) than in those who had received breast milk (90.7 mm Hg).

6.15 A double-blind randomised trial (Hofman et al, 1983) examined the effect of dietary sodium on the blood pressure of 476 full-term new born infants assigned to a low sodium diet (0.1g/4.8 mmol per day) or a normal sodium diet (0.3g/13.4 mmol per day) during the first 6 months of life. At 6 months, a significant difference was observed in systolic blood pressure between the two groups, which was on average 2.1 mm Hg lower in infants fed the low sodium diet compared to infants on the higher sodium diet.

6.16 35% of this cohort (96 participants from the control group and 71 from the low sodium group) were followed up 15 years later (Geleijnse et al, 1996). Systolic and diastolic blood pressures in the intervention group were found to be still significantly lower (3.6/2.2 mm Hg) than in the control group. In contrast with the study groups in the original trial, there were significant differences associated with birth length and weight, maternal systolic blood pressure and maternal education, between the two groups. Subjects in the low sodium group more often reported family history of hypertension, compared with the controls.

Summary and conclusions

6.17 For infants, the sodium levels contained in breast milk are adequate to maintain health. For children, there is a lack of data available regarding the physiological range required for sodium homeostasis. The RNI values for infants and children previously agreed by COMA (DH, 1991) were accepted and used as a basis to set target salt intakes (see Table 2).

6.18 The target average population salt intake, recommended for each age group, does not represent an optimal or ideal consumption level for infants and children but an achievable population goal. Attainment of these levels will require a substantial reduction in current levels of intake.

6.19 There is insufficient evidence to be precise about upper limits for salt intake in relation to cardiovascular risk in children. Rising levels of obesity and lower levels of physical activity increase the potential for occurrence of metabolic syndrome at younger ages and highlight the importance of obesity prevention through lifestyle measures such as a balanced diet and physical activity.

6.20 The evidence of a contribution from salt intake to raised blood pressure in children is limited and it is not clear whether sodium intake in isolation is a factor in the development of hypertension in the young which then tracks into adulthood. More work is needed in this area before firm conclusions can be drawn.

6.21 Further research is needed to assess the level of salt in children's diets, which may influence blood pressure independently of other factors. Nevertheless, it would be inadvisable for children in the UK to become accustomed to the levels of salt intake currently habitual for adults as the evidence suggests long-term consumption of such amounts being potentially harmful in adult life.

7 Research Recommendations

7.1   Development of the evidence base on salt and health is recommended in the following areas:

- effects of habitual intakes of salt on:
  - sodium homeostasis and blood pressure for all age groups, but particularly for infants and children;
  - disease outcomes of the cardiovascular and skeletal system;

- effects of different levels of salt exposure in early life on blood pressure in later life;

- the interrelationship between genetic polymorphisms, metabolic programming, and dietary factors in the regulation of blood pressure and disease outcomes.

British Nutrition Foundation. Salt in the Diet. Briefing Paper, 1994.

Chen Y, Rennie DC, Reeder BA. Age-related association between body mass index and blood pressure: The Humboldt Study. International Journal of Obesity 1995; 19:825-831.

Chinn S, Rona RJ. Prevalence and trends in overweight and obesity in three cross sectional studies of British children, 1974-94. British Medical Journal 2001; 322:24-26.

Cook NR, Cohen J, Herbert P, Taylor JO, Hennekens CH. Implications of small reductions in diastolic blood pressure for primary prevention. Archives of Internal Medicine 1995; 155:701-709.

Corvol P, Persu A, Gimenez-Roqueplo A-P, Jeunemaitre X. Seven lessons from two candidate genes in human essential hypertension. Hypertension 1999; 33:1324-1331.

Cutler JA, Follmann D, Scott Allender P. Randomized trials of sodium reduction: an overview. American Journal of Clinical Nutrition 1997; 65(suppl):643S-51S.

Davey Smith G, Phillips AN. Letters. Intersalt data. British Medical Journal 1997; 315: 484.

Day NE. Letters. Intersalt data. British Medical Journal 1997; 315: 484.

De Garavilla L. Durkot MJ, Ihley TM, Leva N, Francesconi RP. Adverse effects of dietary and furosemide-induced sodium depletion on thermoregulation. Aviation, Space and Environmental Medicine 1990; 61:1012-7.

Denton D, Weisinger R, Mundy NI, Wickings EJ, Dixson A, Moisson P, Pingard AM, Shade R, Carey D, Ardaillou R, Paillard F, Chapman J, Thillet J, Michel JB. The effect of increased salt intake on blood pressure of chimpanzees. Nature Medicine 1995; 1:1009-16.

Department of Environment, Food & Rural Affairs. National Food Survey 2000. TSO, London 2001.

Department of Health. The Annual Report of the Chief Medical Officer of the Department of Health. 2001.

Department of Health. Dietary Reference Values for Food, Energy and Nutrients in the United Kingdom. London: HMSO, 1991. (Report on Health and Social Subjects, No. 41)

Department of Health. Nutritional Aspects of Cardiovascular Disease. London: HMSO, 1994. (Report on Health and Social Subjects, No. 46)

Department of Health. Nutritional Aspects of the Development of Cancer. London: HMSO, 1998. (Report on Health and Social Subjects, No. 48)

Department of Health, Social Services and Public Safety, Northern Ireland. Northern Ireland Health and Social Wellbeing Survey 2001.

Ebrahim S, Davey Smith G. Lowering blood pressure: a systematic review of sustained effects of non-pharmacological interventions. Journal of Public Health Medicine 1998; 20(4):441-448.

Eichberg JW, Shade RE. "Normal" blood pressure in chimpanzees. Journal of Medical Primatology 1987; 16:317-321.

Elliott P, Dyer A, Stamler R, Stamler J. Correcting for regression dilution in INTERSALT. Lancet 1993; 342[8879]:1123.

Elliott P, Stamler J, Nichols R, Dyer AR, Stamler R, Kesteloot H, Marmot M. Intersalt revisited: further analyses of 24 hour sodium excretion and blood pressure within and across populations. Intersalt Cooperative Research Group. British Medical Journal 1996; 312[7041]:1249-53.

Evans CEL, Chughtai AY, Blumsohn A, Giles M, Eastell R. The effect of dietary sodium on calcium metabolism in premenopausal and postmenopausal women. European Journal of Clinical Nutrition 1997; 51:394-399.

Finch S, Doyle W, Lowe C, Bates CJ, Prentice A, Smithers G, Clarke PC. National Diet and Nutrition Survey: people aged 65 years and over. Volume 1: Report of the diet and nutrition survey. TSO, London 1998.

Folkow, B. Physiological aspects of primary hypertension. Physiological Reviews 1982; 62:347-504.

Fomon SJ. Nutrition of normal infants. St Louis, MO, Mosby, 1993.

Francesconi RP, Hubbard RW. Chronic low-sodium diet in rats: Responses to severe heat exposure. Journal of Applied Physiology 1985; 58:152-156.

Francesconi RP, Armstrong LE, Leva N, Moore R, Szlyk PC, Matthew W, Curtis W, Hubbard RW, Askew EW. Endocrinological responses to dietary salt restriction during heat acclimation. Nutritional Needs in Hot Environments: 259-275. Washington DC: National Academy Press, 1993.

Geleijnse JM, Grobbee DE, Hofman A. Sodium and potassium intake and blood pressure change in childhood. British Medical Journal 1990; 300:899-902.

Geleijnse JM, Hofman A, Witteman JCM, Hazebroek AAJM, Valkenburg HA, Grobbee DE. Long-term effects of neonatal sodium restriction on blood pressure. Hypertension 1996; 29(4):913-7.

Gerdts E, Lund-Johansen P, Omvik P. Reproducibility of salt sensitivity testing using a dietary approach in essential hypertension. Journal of Hypertension 1999; 13:375-384.

Ginty F, Flynn A, Cashman KD. The effect of dietary sodium intake on biochemical markers of bone metabolism in young women. British Journal of Nutrition 1998; 79(4):343-50.

Graudal NA, Galloe AM, Garbed P. Effects of sodium restriction on blood pressure, rennin, aldosterone, catecholamines, cholesterols, and triglyceride: a meta-analysis. Journal of American Medical Association 1998; 279[17]:1383-91.

Gregory J, Foster K, Tyler H, Wiseman M. The Dietary and Nutritional Survey of British Adults. HMSO, London 1990.

Gregory J, Lowe S, Bates CJ, Prentice A, Jackson LV, Smithers G, Wenlock, R. Farron M. National Diet and Nutrition Survey: young people aged 4 to 18 years. Volume 1: Report of the diet and nutrition survey. TSO, London 2000.

Gueyffier F et al. Effect of antihypertensive drug treatment on cardiovascular outcomes in women and men. A meta-analysis of individual patient data from randomised controlled trials. Annals of Internal Medicine 1997; 126:761-767.

He J, Tell GS, Tang YC, Mo PS, He GQ. Relation of electrolytes to blood pressure in men. Hypertension 1991; 17:378-385.

He J, Ogden LG, Vupputuri S et al. Dietary sodium intake and subsequent risk of cardiovascular disease in overweight adults. Journal of American Medical Association 1999; 282(21): 2027-34.

Hofman A, Hazelbrock A, Valkenburg HA. A randomized trial of sodium intake and blood pressure in newborn infants. Journal of American Medical Association 1983; 250:370-3.

Hooper L, Bartlett C, Davey Smith G, Ebrahim S. Systematic review of long term effects of advice to reduce dietary salt in adults. British Medical Journal 2002; 325:628.

Hunt SC, Cook NR, Oberman A et al. Angiotensinogen genotype, sodium reduction, weight loss, and prevention of hypertension: trials of hypertension prevention, phase II. Hypertension 1998; 32:393-401.

Infant Formula and Follow-on Formula Regulations 1995, SI 1995 No. 77, as amended. HMSO. London.

Intersalt Cooperative Research Group. Intersalt: an international study of electrolyte excretion and blood pressure. Results for 24 hour urinary sodium and potassium excretion. British Medical Journal 1988; 297:319-28.

John JH, Ziebland S, Yudkin P, Roe LS, Neil HAW. Effects of fruit and vegetable consumption on plasma antioxidant concentrations and blood pressure: a randomised controlled trial. Lancet 2002; 359:1969-74.

Johnson RJ, Herrera-Acosta J, Schreiner GF, Rodriguez-Iturbe B. Subtle acquired renal injury as a mechanism of salt-sensitive hypertension. New England Journal of Medicine 2002; 346:913-923.

Lesniak KT, Dubbert PM. Exercise and hypertension. Current Opinion in Cardiology 2001; 16:356-359.

Levy D, Garrison RJ, Savage DD, Kannel WB, Castelli WP. Left ventricular mass and incidence of coronary heart disease in an elderley cohort: the Framingham Heart Study. Annals of Internal Medicine 1989; 110:101-107.

Liebson PR, Greg A, Grandits G et al. Comparison of five antihypertensive monotherapies and placebo for change in left ventricular mass in patients receiving nutritional-hygienic therapy in the Treatment of Mild Hypertension Study (TOMHS). Circulation 1995; 91:698-706.

Lietz G, Avenell A, Robins SP. Short-term effects of dietary sodium intake on bone metabolism in postmenopausal women measured using urinary deoxypyridinoline excretion. British Journal of Nutrition 1997; 78(1):73-82.

Lin P, Ginty F, Appel L, Svetkey L, Bohannon A, Barclay D, Gannon R, Aickin M. Impact of sodium intake and dietary patterns on biochemical markers of bone and calcium metabolism. Journal of Bone and Mineral Research 2000; 14(S1) M332:S511.

Lurbe E, Alvarez V, Liao Y, Torro I et al. Obesity modifies the relationship between ambulatory blood pressure and natriuresis in children. Blood Pressure Monitoring 2000; 5(5-6):275-80.

MacGregor GA, He FJ. Effect of modest salt reduction on blood pressure: a meta-analysis of randomized trials. Implications for public health. Journal of Human Hypertension 2002; 16:761-770.

MacMahon S, Peto R, Cutler J, Collins R, Sorlie P, Neaton J, Abbot R, Goodwin J, Dyer A, Stamler J. Blood pressure, stroke, and coronary heart disease I. Prolonged differences in blood pressure: prospective observational studies corrected for the regression dilution bias. Lancet 1990; 335:765-774.

Margetts BM, Beilin LJ, Vandongen R, Armstrong BK. Vegetarian diet in mild hypertension: a randomised controlled trial. British Medical Journal 1986; 293:1468-1471.

Marmot MG, Elliott P, Shipley MJ, Dyer AR, Ueshima H, Beevers D, Stamler R, Kesteloot H, Rose G, Stamler J. Alcohol and blood pressure: the INTERSALT study. British Medical Journal 1994; 308:1263-7.

Mattes RD, Falkner B. Salt-sensitivity classification in normotensive adults. Clinical Science 1999; 96:449-459.

McCance RA. Proceedings of the Royal Society of London. Series B-Biological Sciences, Volume 119, 1935-1936. Experimental sodium chloride deficiency in man. Nutrition Review 1990; 48:145-7.

McCarron DA. Letter. New England Journal of Medicine 2001; 344(22):1717.

McParland BE, Goulding A, Campbell AJ. Dietary salt affects biochemical markers of resorption and formation of bone in elderly women. British Medical Journal 1989; 299(6703): 834-5.

McPherson K, Britton A, Causer L. Coronary heart disease: Estimating the impact of changes in risk factors. TSO, London 2002.

Meade TW, Cooper JA, Peart WS. Plasma renin activity and ischemic heart disease. New England Journal of Medicine 1993; 329:616-9.

Midgley JP, Matthew AG, Greenwood CM, Logan AG. Effect of reduced dietary sodium on blood pressure: a meta-analysis of randomized controlled trials. Journal of American Medical Association 1996; 275[20]:1590-7.

Ministry of Agriculture, Fisheries, Food. National Food Survey 1994. HMSO, London 1995.

Morimoto A, Uzu T, Fujii T, Nishimura M, Kuroda S, Nakamura S, Isenaga , Kimura G. Sodium sensitivity and cardiovascular events in patients with essential hypertension. Lancet 1997; 350:1734-1737.

Mulrow CD, Chiquette E, Angel L, Cornell J, Summerbell C, Anagnostelis B, Brand M, Grimm R Jr. Dieting to reduce body weight for controlling hypertension in adults. Cochrane Library 2002; Issue 3.

National Assembly for Wales. Welsh Health Survey 1998. HMSO, 1999.

Nordin BEC, Need AG, Morris HA, Horowitz M. The nature and significance of the relationship between urinary sodium and urinary calcium in women. Journal of Nutrition 1993; 123:1615-1622.

O'Sullivan JJ, Derrick G, Griggs P, Foxall R, Aitkin M, Wren C. Ambulatory blood pressure in children. Archives of Disease in Childhood 1999; 80(6):529-32.

Overlack A, Ruppert M, Kolloch R et al. Divergent hemodynamic and hormonal responses to varying salt intake in normotensive subjects. Hypertension 1993; 22:331-338.

Perry IJ, Beevers DG. Salt intake and stroke: a possible direct effect. Journal of Human Hypertension 1992; 6(1):23-25.

Petitti DB & Freedman D. Letter. New England Journal of Medicine 2001. 344(22):1717.

Poulter NR, Khaw KT, Hopwood BE, Mugambi M, Peart WS, Rose G, Sever PS. The Kenyan Luo migration study: observations on the initiation of a rise in blood pressure. British Medical Journal 1990; 300:967-72.

Power C, Parsons T. Nutritional and other influences in childhood as predictors of adult obesity. Proceeding of the Nutrition Society 2000; 59(2):267-72.

Prospective Studies Collaboration. Age-specific relevance of usual blood pressure to vascular mortality: a meta-analysis of individual data for one million adults in 61 prospective studies. Lancet 2002; 360:1903-13.

Ramsay LE, Willliams B, Johnston GD, MacGregor GA, Poston L, Potter JF, Poulter NR, Russell G. Guidelines for management of hypertension: report of the third working party of the Hypertension Society. Journal of Human Hypertension 1999; 13:569-592.

Rose G. The strategy of preventive medicine. Oxford University Press, 1992.

Ruppert M, Overlack A, Kolloch R, et al. Neurohormonal and metabolic effects of severe and moderate salt restriction in non-obese normotensive adults. Journal of Hypertension 1993; 11:743-9.

Sacks FM, Svetkey LP, Vollmer WM, Appel LJ, Bray GA, Harsha D, Obarzanek E, Conlin PR, Miller ER 3rd, Simons-Morton DG, Karanja N, Lin PH. Effects on blood pressure of reduced dietary sodium and the Dietary Approaches to Stop Hypertension (DASH) diet. DASH-Sodium Collaborative Research Group. New England Journal of Medicine 2001a; 344[1]:3-10.

Sacks FM, Proschan MA, Svetkey LP. Letter. New England Journal of Medicine 2001b; 344(22):1718.

Scientific Advisory Committee on Nutrition 2002. A systematic approach to the evaluation of evidence that relates food and nutrients to health [Online]. Available: http://www.sacn.gov.uk/sacn0202a.pdf

Scottish Office. Eating for health – a diet action plan for Scotland. The Scottish Office Department of Health, Edinburgh, 1996.

Scottish Executive Health Department. The Scottish Health Survey 1998. Joint Surveys Unit, November 2000. TSO.

Sellmeyer DE, Schloetter M, Sebastian A. Potassium citrate prevents increased urine calcium excretion and bone resorption induced by a high sodium chloride diet. Journal of Clinical Endocrinology & Metabolism 2002; 87(5):2008-2012.

Sharma AM, Schattenfroh S, Kribben A, Distler A. Reliability of salt sensitivity testing in normotensive subjects. Klinische Wochenschrift 1989; 67:632-634.

Simons-Morton D, Obarzanek E. Diet and blood pressure in children and adolescents. Pediatric Nephrology 1997; 11:244-249.

Sinaiko AR, Gomez-Marin O, Prineas RJ. Effect of low sodium diet or potassium supplementation on adolescent blood pressure. Hypertension 1993; 21:989-994.

Spitzer A. The role of the kidney in sodium homeostasis during maturation. Kidney International 1982; 21:539-45.

Stamler J, Stamler R, Neaton JD. Blood pressure, systolic and diastolic, and cardiovascular risks. US population data. Archives of Internal Medicine 1993; 153:598-615.

St George IM, Williams SM, Silva PA. Blood pressure level, trend, and variability in Dunedin children. An 8-year study of a single birth cohort. Circulation 1990; 82(5):1675-1680.

Sullivan JM. Salt sensitivity. Definition, conception, methodology, and long-term issues. Hypertension 1991; 17[1 Suppl]:I61-8.

Svetkey LP, Moore TJ, Simons-Morton DG et al. Angiotensinogen genotype and blood pressure response in the DASH study. Journal of Human Hypertension 2001; 19:1949-1956.

Taylor HL, Henschel A, Mickelson O, Keys A. The effect of sodium chloride intake on the work performance of man during exposure to dry heat and experimental heat exhaustion. American Journal of Physiology 1944; 140:439-451.

Tobian L. Hanlon S. High sodium chloride diets injure arteries and raise mortality without changing blood pressure. Hypertension 1990; 15:9003.

Trials of Hypertension Prevention Collaborative Research Group. Effects of weight loss and sodium reduction intervention on blood pressure and hypertension incidence in overweight people with high-normal blood pressure. The Trials of Hypertension Prevention, phase II. Archives of Internal Medicine 1997; 157[6]:657-67.

Tunstall-Pedoe H, Woodward M, Tavendale R, Brook RA, McCluskey MK. Comparison of the prediction by 27 different factors of coronary heart disease and death in men and women of the Scottish heart health study. British Medical Journal (1997); 315:722-729.

Tuomilehto J, Jousilahti P, Rastenyte D, Moltchanov V, Tanskanen A, Pietinen P, Nissinen A. Urinary sodium excretion and cardiovascular mortality in Finland: a prospective study. Lancet 2001; 357[9259]: 848-51.

Weinberger MH, Miller JZ, Luft PC, Grim CE, Fineberg NS. Definitions and characteristics of sodium sensitivity and blood pressure resistance. Hypertension 1986; 8[suppl II]:II127-II 134.

Weinberger MH, Fineberg NS. Sodium and volume sensitivity of blood pressure: age and pressure change over time. Hypertension 1991; 18:67-71.

Weinberger MH, Fineberg NS, Fineberg SE, Weinberger M. Salt sensitivity, pulse pressure, and death in normal and hypertensive humans. Hypertension 2001; 37[2]: 429-32.

Wheelock V, Hobbiss A. All you ever wanted to know about salt but were afraid to ask. Verner Wheelock Associates. Skipton, Yorkshire 1999.

Whelton PK, Appel LJ, Espeland MA, et al. Sodium reduction and weight loss in the treatment of hypertension in older persons: a randomised controlled trial of nonpharmacologic interventions in the elderly (TONE): TONE Collaborative Research Group. Journal of the American Medical Association 1998; 279:839-846.

Whelton SP, Chin A, Xin X, He J. Effect of aerobic exercise on blood pressure: A meta-analysis of randomized, controlled trials. Annals of Internal Medicine 2002; 136:493-503.

Wilson AC, Forsyth JS, Greene SA, Irvine L, Hau C. Relation of infant diet to childhood health: seven year follow up of cohort of children in Dundee infant feeding study. British Medical Journal 1998; 316:21-5.

Wilson DK, Bayer L, Krishnamoorthy JS, Ampey-Thornhill G, Nicholson SC, Sica DA. The prevalence of salt sensitivity in an African-American adolescent population. Ethnicity and Disease 1999; 9(3):350-8.

Xin X, He J, Frontini MG, Ogden LG, Motsamai OI, Whelton PK. Effects of alcohol reduction on blood pressure: a meta-analysis of randomised controlled trials. Hypertension 2001; 38(5):1112-7.

Yamori Y, Nara Y, Mizushima S, Sawamura M, Horie R. Nutritional factors for stroke and major cardiovascular diseases: international epidemiological comparison of dietary prevention. Health reports (1994); 6:22-27.

Zoccali C, Mallamaci F, Cuzzola F, Leonardis D. Reproducibility of the response to short-term low salt intake in essential hypertension. Journal of Hypertension 1996; 14:1455-1459.

Annex 1

Responses Received by SACN to the Call for Submissions on Salt

A call to submit evidence to the Salt Subgroup of SACN was placed on the website on 17 October 2001; deadline for receipt of submissions was 3 December 2001.

Responses were received from the following organisations:

1. Consensus Action on Salt and Health

2. The Salt Manufacturers' Association

3. Food & Drink Federation

4. Cardiovascular Research Institute, University of Leicester

5. J Sainsbury plc

6. Verner Wheelock Associates

7. British Retail Consortium

8. Safeway Stores plc

9. Co-operative Group

All the responses can be viewed in full at the SACN website (www.sacn.gov.uk)

Annex 2

Working Procedures

Identification of relevant studies since 1994

The framework for risk assessment developed by SACN (2002) was used to identify and evaluate available evidence.

In response to submissions received from interested parties, the specific areas for which further information was sought and the search terms that were used are outlined in the table below. The search terms were used alone, combined with hypertension/blood pressure, or in various other combinations.

TOPIC	SEARCH TERMS
Salt deprivation, acute adaptation, conservation	salt/sodium deprivation salt/sodium adaptation adaptation to low sodium intake intake/low salt intake acute adaptive response salt/sodium conservation hypertension/blood pressure
Sodium reduction/restriction	sodium/salt reduction sodium/salt restriction
Sodium balance	sodium balance
Salt sensitivity	salt/sodium sensitivity salt/sodium loading
Effect of chloride	chloride non-chloride/nonchloride sodium salts
Renal handling of sodium in children	renal physiology renal physiology in children renal handling of sodium/salt in children renal effects of sodium/salt in children

Medline was the main source for identification of studies. The Cochrane Database for Systematic Reviews was also checked. In addition, papers listed in the submissions from interested parties and references cited in other papers were obtained.

Responses received to draft report on Salt and Health

The draft report was placed on the SACN website on 4 November 2002. Interested parties were invited to submit comments on the draft report by 3 January 2003.

Responses were received from the following organisations & individuals:

1. British Dietetic Association

2. British Frozen Food Federation

3. British Nutrition Foundation

4. British Retail Consortium

5. Cochrane Heart Group

6. Consensus Action on Salt and Health

7. Co-operative Group

8. Food Commission

9. Food & Drink Federation

10. Hooper L, Bartlett C, Davey Smith G, Ebrahim S

11. Inside Story

12. Institute of Food Science & Technology (UK)

13. Intercollegiate Group on Nutrition

14. LoSalt

15. Macnair A

16. McGee E

17. Meat & Livestock Commission

18. Medical Research Council, Human Nutrition Research

19. National Heart Forum

20. National Osteoporosis Society

21. Nutrition Society

22. Sainsbury's

23. Salt Institute

24. Salt Manufacturers' Association

25. Scottish Consumer Council

26. Socialist Health Association

27. Snacks, Nuts & Crisps Manufacturers Association

28. Stroke Association

28 responses were received to the draft report. 15 respondents were in agreement with the conclusions of the draft report; 2 respondents agreed with parts of the draft report; 4 respondents raised specific points but did not state whether they agreed with the main conclusions; and 7 respondents did not agree with the conclusions. The responses can be viewed, in full, on the SACN website (www.sacn.gov.uk).

Papers considered by the Salt Subgroup

Alam S, Johnson AG. A meta-analysis of randomised controlled trials (RCT) among healthy normotensive and essential hypertensive elderly patients to determine the effect of high salt (NaCl) diet of blood pressure. Journal of Human Nutrition Hypertension 1999; 13[6]:367-74.

Al-Dahhan J, Haycock GB, Chantler C, Stimmler L. Sodium homeostasis in term and preterm neonates. I. Renal aspects. Archives of Disease in Childhood 1983; 58:335-42.

Al-Dahhan J, Haycock GB, Chantler C, Stimmler L. Sodium homeostasis in term and preterm neonates. II. Gastrointestinal aspects. Archives of Disease in Childhood 1983; 58:343-5.

Al-Dahhan J, Haycock GB, Nichol B, Chantler C, Stimmler L. Sodium homeostasis in term and preterm neonates. III. Effect of salt supplementation. Archives of Disease in Childhood 1984; 59:945-50.

Alderman M. Letter. New England Journal of Medicine 2001; 344(22):1716.

Alderman MH, Cohen H, Madhavan S. Dietary sodium intake and mortality: the National Health and Nutrition Examination Survey. Lancet 1998; 351:781-785.

Alderman MH, Madhavan S, Cohen H, Sealey JE, Laragh JH. Low urinary sodium is associated with greater risk of myocardial infarction among treated hypertensive men. Hypertension 1995; 25:1144-52.

Allsopp AJ, Sutherland R, Wood P, Wootton SA, The effect of sodium balance on sweat sodium secretion and plasma aldosterone concentration, European Journal of Applied Physiology 1998; 78(6):516-21.

Appel LJ, Moore TJ, Obarzanek E, Vollmer WM, Svetkey LP, Sacks FM, Bray GA, Vogt TM, Cutler JA, Windhauser MM, Lin PH, Karanja N. A clinical trial of the effects of dietary patterns on blood pressure. DASH Collaborative Research Group. New England Journal of Medicine 1997; 336[16]: 1117-24.

Armstrong LE, Hubbard RW, Askew EW et al. Responses to moderate and low sodium diets during exercise-heat acclimation. International Journal of Sport Nutrition 1993; 3:207-221.

Aristimuno GG, Foster TA, Berenson GS, Akman D. Subtle electrocardiographic changes in children with high levels of blood pressure. American Journal of Cardiology 1984; 54(10):1272-6.

Bajckal M, Primatesta P, Prior G. Health Survey for England 2001. TSO, London 2003.

Barba G, Cappuccio FP, Russo L et al. Renal function and blood pressure response to dietary salt restriction in normotensive men. Hypertension 1996; 27:1160-1164.

Barden AE, Vandongen R, Beilin LJ, Margetts B, Rogers P. Potassium supplementation does not lower blood pressure in normotensive women. Journal of Human Hypertension 1986; 4:339-343.

Beil AH, Schmieder RE. Salt intake as a determinant of cardiac hypertrophy. Blood Press Supplement 1995; 2:30-4.

Bingham SA, Cummings JH. The use of creatinine output as a check on the completeness of 24h urine collections. Human Nutrition: Clinical Nutrition 1985; 39c:343-353.

Bingham SA, Williams R, Cole TJ, Price CP, Cummings JH. Reference values for analytes of 24-h urine collections known to be complete. Annals of Clinical Biochemistry 1988; 25:610-9.

British Nutrition Foundation. Salt in the Diet. Briefing Paper, 1994.

Bueva A, Guignard JP. Renal function in preterm neonates. Pediatric Research 1994; 36:572-7.

Cappuccio FP, Kalaitzidis R, Duneclift S, Eastwood JB. Unravelling the links between calcium excretion, salt intake, hypertension, kidney stones and bone metabolism. Journal of Nephrology 2000; 13:169-177.

Cappuccio FP, MacGregor GA. Does potassium supplementation lower blood pressure? A meta-analysis of published trials. Journal of Human Hypertension 1991; 9:465-73.

Cappuccio FP, Markandu ND, Carney C, Sagnella GA, Macgregor GA. Double-blind randomised trial of modest salt restriction in older people. Lancet 1997; 350:850-4.

Chen Y, Rennie DC, Reeder BA. Age-related association between body mass index and blood pressure: The Humboldt Study. International Journal of Obesity 1995; 19:825-831.

Chevalier RL. The moth and the aspen tree: sodium in early postnatal development. Kidney International 2001; 59:1617-1625.

Chinn S, Rona RJ. Prevalence and trends in overweight and obesity in three cross sectional studies of British children, 1974-94. British Medical Journal 2001; 322:24-26.

Chiolero A, Maillard M, Nussberger J, Brunner H-R & Burnier M. Proximal sodium reabsorption: an independent determinant of blood pressure response to salt. Hypertension 2000; 36: 631-7.

Chiolero A, Wurzner G, Burnier M. Renal determinants of the salt sensitivity of blood pressure. Nephrology Dialysis Transplantation 2001; 16:452-458.

Chobanian AV, Hill M. National Heart, Lung, and Blood Institute Workshop on Sodium and Blood Pressure: A critical review of current scientific evidence. Hypertension 2000; 35:858-863.

Chrysant GS, Bakir S, Oparil S. Dietary salt reduction in hypertension — what is the evidence and why is it still controversial? Progress in Cardiovascular Diseases 1999; 42(1):23-38.

Cohen AJ, Roe FJC. Review of risk factors for osteoporosis with particular reference to a possible aetiological role of dietary salt. Food and Chemical Toxicology 2000; 38:237-253.

Conlin PR, Chow D, Miler ER III, et al. The effect of dietary patterns on blood pressure control in hypertensive patients: results from the Dietary Approaches to Stop Hypertension (DASH) trial. American Journal of Hypertension 2000; 13:949-955.

Conn JW. Aldosteronism in man: Some clinical and climatological aspects. Part I. Journal of American Medical Association 1963; 183:775-781.

Convertino VA, Keil LC, Bernauer EM, Greenleaf JE. Plasma volume, osmolality, vasopressin, and renin activity during graded exercise in man. Journal of Applied Physiology 1981; 50:123-8.

Cook NR, Cohen J, Herbert P, Taylor JO, Hennekens CH. Implications of small reductions in diastolic blood pressure for primary prevention. Archives of Internal Medicine 1995; 155:701-709.

Cooper R, Liu K, Trevisan M, Miller W, Stamler J. Urinary sodium excretion and blood pressure in children: absence of a reproducible association. Hypertension 1983; 5:135-9.

Cooper R, Soltero I, Liu K, Berkson D, Levinson S, Stamler J. The association between urinary sodium excretion and blood pressure in children. Circulation 1980; 62:97-104.

Corvol P, Persu A, Gimenez-Roqueplo A-P, Jeunemaitre X. Seven lessons from two candidate genes in human essential hypertension. Hypertension 1999; 33:1324-1331.

Costill DL, Branam G, Fink W, Nelson R. Exercise induced sodium conservation: changes in plasma renin and aldosterone. Medicine and Science in Sports and Exercise 1976; 8:209-13.

Crystal SR, Bernstein IL. Infant salt preference and mother's morning sickness. Appetite 1998; 30:297-307.

Crystal SR, Bernstein IL. Morning sickness: impact on offspring salt preference. Appetite 1995; 25:231-40.

Cutler JA, Follmann D, Scott Allender P. Randomized trials of sodium reduction: an overview. American Journal of Clinical Nutrition 1997; 65(suppl):643S-51S.

Dahl LK. Salt intake and salt need. New England Journal of Medicine 1958; 258(23):1205-8.

Dahl LK. Salt intake and salt need. New England Journal of Medicine 1958; 258:1152-1157.

Davey Smith G, Phillips AN. Letters. Intersalt data. British Medical Journal 1997; 315: 484.

Day NE. Letters. Intersalt data. British Medical Journal 1997; 315: 484.

De Garavilla L, Durkot MJ, Ihley TM, Leva N, Francesconi RP. Adverse effects of dietary and furosemide-induced sodium depletion on thermoregulation. Aviation Space, and Environmental Medicine 1990; 61:1012-7.

Denton D, Weisinger R, Mundy NI, Wickings EJ, Dixson A, Moisson P, Pingard AM, Shade R, Carey D, Ardaillou R, Paillard F, Chapman J, Thillet J, Michel JB. The effect of increased salt intake on blood pressure of chimpanzees. Nature Medicine 1995; 1:1009-16.

Department of Environment, Food & Rural Affairs. National Food Survey 2000. TSO, London 2001.

Department of Health. The Annual Report of the Chief Medical Officer of the Department of Health. 2001.

Department of Health. Dietary Reference Values for Food, Energy and Nutrients in the United Kingdom. London: HMSO, 1991. (Report on Health and Social Subjects, No. 41)

Department of Health. Nutritional Aspects of Cardiovascular Disease. London: HMSO, 1994. (Report on Health and Social Subjects, No. 46)

Department of Health. Nutritional Aspects of the Development of Cancer. London: HMSO, 1998. (Report on Health and Social Subjects, No. 48)

Department of Health, Social Services and Public Safety, Northern Ireland. Northern Ireland Health and Social Wellbeing Survey 2001.

De Wardener HE, MacGregor GA. Harmful effects of dietary salt in addition to hypertension. Journal of Human Hypertension 2002; 16:213-223.

De Wardener HE. Salt reduction and cardiovascular risk: the anatomy of a myth. Journal of Human Hypertension 1999; 13:1-4.

Dean RFA, McCance RA. The renal responses of infants and adults to the administration of hypertonic solutions of sodium chloride and urea. Journal of Physiology (Lond) 1949; 109:81-97

Denton D, Weisinger R, Mundy NI et al. The effect of increased salt intake on blood pressure of chimpanzees. Nature Medicine 1995; 1:1009-16.

Ebrahim S, Davey Smith G. Lowering blood pressure: a systematic review of sustained effects of non-pharmacological interventions. Journal of Public Health Medicine 1998; 20(4):441-448.

Eichberg JW, Shade RE. "Normal" blood pressure in chimpanzees. Journal of Medical Primatology 1987; 16:317-321.

Elliott P, Dyer A, Stamler R, Stamler J. Correcting for regression dilution in INTERSALT. Lancet 1993; 342[8879]:1123.

Elliott P, Stamler J, Nichols R, Dyer AR, Stamler R, Kesteloot H, Marmot M. Intersalt revisited: further analyses of 24 hour sodium excretion and blood pressure within and across populations. Intersalt Cooperative Research Group. British Medical Journal 1996; 312[7041]:1249-53.

Erens B, Primatesta P Eds. Health Survey for England, Cardiovascular Disease 1998. TSO, London.

Evans CEL, Chughtai AY, Blumsohn A, Giles M, Eastell R. The effect of dietary sodium on calcium metabolism in premenopausal and postmenopausal women. European Journal of Clinical Nutrition 1997; 51:394-399.

Falkner B, Michel S. Blood pressure response to sodium in children and adolescents. American Journal of Clinical Nutrition 1997; 65 (suppl):681S-21S.

Faust HS. Effects of drinking water and total sodium intake on blood pressure. American Journal of Clinical Nutrition 1982; 35:1459-67.

Finch S, Doyle W, Lowe C, Bates CJ, Prentice A, Smithers G, Clarke PC. National Diet and Nutrition Survey: people aged 65 years and over. Volume 1: Report of the diet and nutrition survey. TSO, London 1998.

Fodor JG, Whitmore B, Leenen F, Larochelle P. Recommendations on dietary salt. Canadian Medical Association Journal 1999; 160(9): S29-S34.

Folkow, B. Physiological aspects of primary hypertension. Physiological Review 1982; 62:347-504.

Fomon SJ. Nutrition of normal infants. St Louis, MO, Mosby, 1993.

Francesconi RP and Hubbard RW. Chronic low-sodium diet in rats: Responses to severe heat exposure. Journal of Applied Physiology 1985; 58:152-156.

Francesconi RP, Armstrong LE, Leva N, Moore R, Szlyk PC, Matthew W, Curtis W, Hubbard RW, Askew EW. Endocrinological responses to dietary salt restriction during heat acclimation. Nutritional Needs in Hot Environments: 259-275. Washington DC: National Academy Press, 1993

Geleijnse JM, Grobbee DE, Hofman A. Sodium and potassium intake and blood pressure change in childhood. British Medical Journal 1990; 300:899-902.

Geleijnse JM, Hofman A, Witteman JCM, Hazebroek AAJM, Valkenburg HA, Grobbee DE. Long-term effects of neonatal sodium restriction on blood pressure. Hypertension 1996; 29:913-7.

Gerdts E, Lund-Johansen P, Omvik P. Reproducibility of salt sensitivity testing using a dietary approach in essential hypertension. Journal of Hypertension 1999; 13:375-384.

Gillman MW, Oliveria SA, Moore LL, Ellison RC. Inverse association of dietary calcium with systolic blood pressure in young children. Journal of American Medical Association 1992; 267:2340-3.

Gillum RF, Elmer PJ, Prineas RJ. Changing sodium intake in children. The Minneapolis Children's Blood Pressure Study. Hypertension 1981; 3:698-703.

Ginty F, Flynn A, Cashman KD. The effect of dietary sodium intake on biochemical markers of bone metabolism in young women. British Journal of Nutrition 1998; 79(4):343-50.

Gomez RA, Norwood VF. Developmental consequences of the renin-angiotensin system. American Journal of Kidney Disease 1995; 26:409-31.

Graudal NA, Galloe AM, Garbed P. Effects of sodium restriction on blood pressure, rennin, aldosterone, catecholamines, cholesterols, and triglyceride: a meta-analysis. Journal of American Medical Association 1998; 279[17]:1383-91.

Gregory J, Foster K, Tyler H, Wiseman M. The Dietary and Nutritional Survey of British Adults. HMSO, London 1990.

Gregory, J., Lowe, S., Bates, C.J., Prentice, A., Jackson, L.V., Smithers, G., Wenlock, R. and Farron, M. National Diet and Nutrition Survey: young people aged 4 to 18 years Volume 1: Report of the diet and nutrition survey. The Stationery Office, London 2000.

Grim CE, Wilson TW. Salt, slavery and survival: physiological principles underlying the hypothesis of salt-sensitive hypertension in western hemisphere blacks. In Fray JCS, Douglas JG, eds. Pathophysiology of hypertension in Blacks. New York, NY: Oxford University Press; 1993:25-49.

Grimm RH Jr, Neaton JD, Elmer PJ et al. The influence of oral potassium chloride on blood pressure in hypertensive men on a low-sodium diet. New England Journal of Medicine 1990; 322:569-74.

Gueyffier F et al. Effect of antihypertensive drug treatment on cardiovascular outcomes in women and men. A meta-analysis of individual patient data from randomised controlled trials. Annals of Internal Medicine 1997; 126:761-767.

Hargreaves M, Morgan TO, Snow R, Guerin M. Exercise tolerance in the heat on low and normal salt intakes. Clinical Science 1989; 76:553-557.

He J, Tell GS, Tang YC, Mo PS, He GQ. Relation of electrolytes to blood pressure in men. Hypertension 1991; 17:378-385.

He J, Odgen LG, Vupputuri S, Bazzano LA, Loria C, Whelton PK. Dietary sodium intake and subsequent risk of cardiovascular disease in overweight adults. Journal of American Medical Association 1999; 282:2027-2034.

He FJ, Markandu ND, Sagnella GA, MacGregor GA. Effect of salt intake on renal excretion of water in humans. Hypertension 2001;38:317-20.

Heino T, Kallio K, Jokinen et al. Sodium intake of 1 to 5-year old children: the STRIP project. Acta Paediatrica 2000; 89:406-410.

Hofman A, Hazelbrock A, Valkenburg HA. A randomized trial of sodium intake and blood pressure in newborn infants. Journal of American Medical Association 1983; 250:370-3.

Hofman A, Valkenburg HA, Vaandroger GT. Increased blood pressure in school children related to high sodium levels in drinking water. Journal of Epidemiology and Community Health 1980; 34:179-81.

Hooper L, Bartlett C, Davey Smith G, Ebrahim S. Systematic review of long term effects of advice to reduce dietary salt in adults. British Medical Journal 2002; 325:628.

Hunt SC, Cook NR, Oberman A et al. Angiotensinogen genotype, sodium reduction, weight loss, and prevention of hypertension: trials of hypertension prevention, phase II. Hypertension 1998; 32:393-401.

Huxley RR, Law CM, Shiell AW. The role of size at birth and postnatal catch-up growth in determining systolic blood pressure: a systematic review of the literature. Journal of Human Hypertension 2000 Jul; 18(7): 815-31

Infant Formula and Follow-on Formula Regulations 1995, SI 1995 No. 77, as amended. HMSO. London.

Intersalt Cooperative Research Group. Intersalt: an international study of electrolyte excretion and blood pressure. Results for 24 hour urinary sodium and potassium excretion. British Medical Journal 1988; 297:319-28.

John JH, Ziebland S, Yudkin P, Roe LS, Neil HAW. Effects of fruit and vegetable consumption on plasma antioxidant concentrations and blood pressure: a randomised controlled trial. Lancet 2002; 359:1969-74.

Johnson RJ, Herrera-Acosta J, Schreiner GF, Rodriguez-Iturbe B. Subtle acquired renal injury as a mechanism of salt-sensitive hypertension. New England Journal of Medicine 2002; 346:913-923.

Jose PA, Fildes RD, Gomez RA, Chevalier RL, Robillard JE. Neonatal renal function and physiology. Current Opinion in Pediatrics 1994; 6:172-177.

Kant AK, Schatzkin A. Graubard BI, Schairer C. A prospective study of diet quality and mortality in women. Journal of American Medical Association 2000; 283:2109-2115.

Klabunde RE. 2001. Renin-Angiotensin system. [Online]. Available: http://www.oucom.ohiou.edu/cvphysiology/ BP015.htm.

Kotchen TA, Kotchen JM. Dietary sodium and blood pressure: interactions with other nutrients. American Journal of Clinical Nutrition 1997; 65(suppl):708S-11S.

Kotchen TA, McCarron DA. Dietary electrolytes and blood pressure. A statement for healthcare professionals from the American Heart Association Nutrition Committee. Circulation 1998; 98:613-617.

Kumanyika SK, Cutler JA. Dietary sodium reduction: Is there cause for concern? 1997. Journal of the American College of Nutrition; 16(3):192-203.

Kurokawa K. Tubuglomerular feedback: its physiological and pathophysiological significance. Kidney International 1998; 54 (suppl 67):S71-S74.

Law CM, Shiell AW. Is blood pressure inversely related to birth weight? The strength of evidence from a systematic review of the literature. Journal of Human Hypertension 1996; 14(8): 935-41.

Lesniak KT, Dubbert PM. Exercise and hypertension. Current Opinion in Cardiology 2001; 16:356-359.

Levy D, Garrison RJ, Savage DD, Kannel WB, Castelli WP. Left ventricular mass and incidence of coronary heart disease in an elderley cohort: the Framingham Heart Study. Annals of Internal Medicine 1989; 110:101-107.

Liebman M, Chopin LF, Carter E et al. Factors related to blood pressure in a biracial adolescent female population. Hypertension 1986; 8:843-50.

Liebson PR, Grandits GA, Dianzumba S, Prineas RJ, Grimm RH, Neaton JD, Stamler J. Comparison of five antihypertensive monotherapies and placebo for change in left ventricular mass in patients receiving nutritional-hygienic therapy in the Treatment of Mild Hypertension Study (TOMHS). Circulation 1995; 91: 698-706.

Lietz G, Avenell A, Robins SP. Short-term effects of dietary sodium intake on bone metabolism in postmenopausal women measured using urinary deoxypyridinoline excretion. British Journal of Nutrition 1997; 78(1):73-82.

Lin P, Ginty F, Appel L, Svetkey L, Bohannon A, Barclay D, Gannon R, Aickin M. Impact of sodium intake and dietary patterns on biochemical markers of bone and calcium metabolism. Journal of Bone and Mineral Research 2000; 14(S1) M332:S511.

Liu K, Cooper RS, Soltero I, Stamler J. Variability in 24-hour urine sodium excretion in children. Hypertension 1979;1:631-6.

Lowder SC, Brown RD. Hypertension corrected by discontinuing chronic sodium bicarbonate ingestion. American Journal of Medicine (1975); 58:272.

Lucas A, Morley R, Cole TJ, Gore SM. A randomised multicentre study of human milk versus formula and later development in preterm infants. Archives of Disease in Childhood, Fetal and Neonatal Edition 1994; 70[2]:F141-6.

Lucas A, Morley R, Hudson GJ, Bamford MF, Boon A, Crowle P, Dossetor JF, Pearse R. Early sodium intake and later blood pressure in preterm infants. Archives of Disease in Childhood 1988; 63[6]:656-7.

Luft FC, Rankin LI, Bloch R, Weyman AE, Willis LR, Murray RH, Grim CE, Weinberger MH. Cardiovascular and humoral responses to extremes of sodium intake in normal black and white men. Circulation 1979; 60:697-706.

Lurbe E, Alvarez V, Liao Y, Torro I et al. Obesity modifies the relationship between ambulatory blood pressure and natriuresis in children. Blood Press Monitor 2000; 5(5-6):275-80.

MacGregor GA, He FJ. Effect of modest salt reduction on blood pressure: a meta-analysis of randomized trials. Implications for public health. Journal of Human Hypertension 2002; 16:761-770.

MacMahon S, Peto R, Cutler J, Collins R, Sorlie P, Neaton J, Abbot R, Goodwin J, Dyer A, Stamler J. Blood pressure, stroke, and coronary heart disease I. Prolonged differences in blood pressure: prospective observational studies corrected for the regression dilution bias. Lancet 1990; 335:765-774.

Margetts BM, Beilin LJ, Armstrong BK, Rouse IL, Vandongen R, Croft KD, McMurchie EJ. Blood pressure and dietary polyunsaturated and saturated fats: a controlled trial. Clinical Science 1985; 69:165-175.

Margetts BM, Beilin LJ, Vandongen R, Armstrong BK. A randomized controlled trial of the effect of dietary fibre on blood pressure. Clinical Science 1987; 72:343-350.

Margetts BM, Beilin LJ, Vandongen R, Armstrong BK. Vegetarian diet in mild hypertension: a randomised controlled trial. British Medical Journal 1986; 293:1468-1471.

Marmot MG, Elliott P, Shipley MJ, Dyer AR, Ueshima H, Beevers D, Stamler R, Kesteloot H, Rose G, Stamler J. Alcohol and blood pressure: the INTERSALT study. British Medical Journal 1994; 308:1263-7.

Mattes RD, Falkner B. Salt-sensitivity classification in normotensive adults. Clinical Science 1999; 96:449-459.

McCance RA. Proceedings of the Royal Society of London. Series B—Biological Sciences, Volume 119, 1935-1936: Experimental sodium chloride deficiency in man. Nutrition Review 1990; 48:145-7.

McCarron DA. Letter. New England Journal of Medicine 2001; 344(22):1717.

McParland BE, Goulding A, Campbell AJ. Dietary salt affects biochemical markers of resorption and formation of bone in elderly women. British Medical Journal 1989; 299(6703):834-5.

McPherson K, Britton A, Causer L. Coronary heart disease: Estimating the impact of changes in risk factors. TSO, London 2002.

Meade TW, Cooper JA, Peart WS. Plasma renin activity and ischemic heart disease. New England Journal of Medicine 1993; 329:616-9.

Midgley JP, Matthew AG, Greenwood CMT, Logan AG. Effect of reduced dietary sodium on blood pressure: a meta-analysis of randomized controlled trials. Journal of American Medical Association 1996; 275: 1590-97.

Miller JZ, Daugherty SA, Weinberger MH, Grim CE, Christian JC, Lang CL. Blood pressure response to dietary sodium restriction in normotensive adults. Hypertension 1983;5:790-795.

Ministry of Agriculture, Fisheries, Food. National Food Survey 1994. HMSO, London 1995.

Morimoto A, Uzu T, Fujii T, Nishimura M, Kuroda S, Nakamura S, Isenaga , Kimura G. Sodium sensitivity and cardiovascular events in patients with essential hypertension. Lancet 1997; 350:1734-1737.

Mulrow CD, Chiquette E, Angel L, Cornell J, Summerbell C, Anagnostelis B, Brand M, Grimm R Jr. Dieting to reduce body weight for controlling hypertension in adults. Cochrane Library 2002; Issue 3.

National Assembly for Wales. Welsh Health Survey 1998. HMSO, 1999.

Need AG, Morris HA, Cleghorn DB, De Nichilo D, Horowitz M, Nordin BE. Effect of salt restriction on hydroxyproline excretion in postmenopausal women. Archives of Internal Medicine 1991; 151(4):757-9.

Nordin BEC, Need AG, Morris HA, Horowitz M. The nature and significance of the relationship between urinary sodium and urinary calcium in women. Journal of Nutrition 1993; 123:1615-1622.

O'Sullivan JJ, Derrick G, Griggs P, Foxall R, Aitkin M, Wren C. Ambulatory blood pressure in children. Archives of Disease in Childhood 1999; 80(6):529-32.

Overlack A, Ruppert M, Kolloch R et al. Divergent hemodynamic and hormonal responses to varying salt intake in normotensive subjects. Hypertension 1993; 22:331-338.

Perry IJ, Beevers DG. Salt intake and stroke: a possible direct effect. Journal of Human Hypertension 1992; 6(1):23-5.

Petitti DB & Freedman D. Letter. New England Journal of Medicine 2001. 344(22):1717.

Pomeranz A, Dolfin T, Korzets Z, Eliakim A, Wolach B. Increase sodium concentrations in drinking water increase blood pressure in neonates. Journal of Hypertension 2002; 20:203-207.

Poulter NR, Khaw KT, Hopwood BE, Mugambi M, Peart WS, Rose G, Sever PS. The Kenyan Luo migration study: observations on the initiation of a rise in blood pressure. British Medical Journal 1990; 300:967-72.

Power C, Parsons T. Nutritional and other influences in childhood as predictors of adult obesity. Proceeding of the Nutrition Society 2000; 59(2):267-72.

Powles JW, Hopper JL, Macaskill GT, Ktenas D. Blood pressure in subjects from rural Greece, comparing individuals migrating to Melbourne, Australia with non-migrant relatives. Journal of Human Hypertension 1993; 7:419-428

Prescott SL, Jenner DA, Beilin LJ, Margetts BM, Vandongen R. A randomized controlled trial of the effect on blood pressure of dietary non-meat protein versus meat protein in normotensive omnivores. Clinical Science 1988; 74:665-672.

Prospective Studies Collaboration. Age-specific relevance of usual blood pressure to vascular mortality: a meta-analysis of individual data for one million adults in 61 prospective studies. Lancet 2002; 360:1903-13.

Ramsay LE, Williams B, Johnston GD, MacGregor GA, Poston L, Potter JF, Poulter NR, Russell G. Guidelines for management of hypertension: report of the third working party of the Hypertension Society. Journal of Human Hypertension 1999; 13:569-592.

Reddy KA, Marth EH. Reducing the sodium content of foods: A review. Journal of Food Protection 1991; 54(2):138-150.

Rose G. The strategy of preventive medicine. Oxford University Press, 1992.

Ross B, Cowett RM, Oh W. Renal functions of low birth weight infants during the first two months of life. Pediatric Research 1977;11:1162-4.

Ruppert M, Overlack A, Kolloch R, et al. Neurohormonal and metabolic effects of severe and moderate salt restriction in non-obese normotensive adults. Journal of Human Hypertension 1993; 11:743-9.

Sacks FM, Svetkey LP, Vollmer WM, Appel LJ, Bray GA, Harsha D, Obarzanek E, Conlin PR, Miller ER 3rd, Simons-Morton DG, Karanja N, Lin PH. Effects on blood pressure of reduced dietary sodium and the Dietary Approaches to Stop Hypertension (DASH) diet. DASH-Sodium Collaborative Research Group. New England Journal of Medicine 2001; 344[1]: 3-10.

Sacks FM, Proschan MA, Svetkey LP. Letter. New England Journal of Medicine 2001; 344(22):1718.

Schmieder RE, Messerli FH, Garavaglia GE, Nunez BD. Dietary Salt Intake: A determinant of cardiac involvement in essential hypertension. Circulation 1988; 78(4): 951-956.

Scientific Advisory Committee on Nutrition 2002. A systematic approach to the evaluation of evidence that relates food and nutrients to health [Online]. Available: www.sacn.gov.uk/sacn0202a.pdf

Scottish Executive Health Department. The Scottish Health Survey 1998. Joint Surveys Unit, November 2000. TSO.

Scottish Office. Eating for health – a diet action plan for Scotland. The Scottish Office Department of Health, Edinburgh, 1996.

Sellmeyer DE, Schloetter M, Sebastian A. Potassium citrate prevents increase urine calcium excretion and bone resorption induced by a high sodium chloride diet. The Journal of Clinical Endocrinology and Metabolism; 87(5):2008-2012.

Sharma AM, Schattenfroh S, Kribben A, Distler A. Reliability of salt sensitivity testing in normotensive subjects. Klinische Wochenshrift 1989; 67:632-634.

Simons-Morton DG, Orbazanek E. Diet and blood pressure in children and adolescents. Pediatric Nephrology 1997; 11:244-249.

Sinaiko A, Gomez-Marin O, Prineas RJ. Effect of low sodium diet or potassium supplementation on adolescent blood pressure. Hypertension 1993; 21:989-994.

Singhal A, Cole TJ, Lucas A. Early nutrition in preterm infants and later blood pressure: two cohorts after randomised trials. Lancet 357[9254], 413-9. 2001.

Spitzer A. The role of the kidney in sodium homeostasis during maturation. Kidney International 1982; 21:539-45.

Stamler J, Stamler R, Neaton JD. Blood pressure, systolic and diastolic, and cardiovascular risks. US population data. Archives of Internal Medicine 1993; 153:598-615.

St George IM, Williams SM, Silva PA. Blood pressure level, trend, and variability in Dunedin children. An 8-year study of a single birth cohort. Circulation 1990; 82(5):1675-1680.

Strauss MB, Lamdin E, Smith WP, Bleifer DJ. Surfeit and deficit of sodium. Archives of Internal Medicine 1958:102:527-536.

Sullivan JM. Salt sensitivity. Definition, conception, methodology, and long-term issues. Hypertension 1991; 17[1 Suppl]:161-8.

Svetkey LP, Moore TJ, Simons-Morton DG et al. Angiotensinogen genotype and blood pressure response in the DASH study. Journal of Human Hypertension 2001; 19:1949-1956.

Taylor HL, Henschel A, Mickelson O, Keys A. The effect of sodium chloride intake on the work performance of man during exposure to dry heat and experimental heat exhaustion. American Journal of Physiology, 1944; 140:439-451.

Tobian L, Hanlon S. High sodium chloride diets injure arteries and raise mortality without changing blood pressure. Hypertension 1990; 15:9003.

Trials of Hypertension Prevention Collaborative Research Group. Effect of weight loss and sodium reduction intervention on blood pressure and hypertension incidence in overweight people with high-normal blood pressure. The Trials of Hypertension Prevention, Phase II. Archives of Internal Medicine 1997; 157:657-67.

Tunstall-Pedoe H, Woodward M, Tavendale R, Brook RA, McCluskey MK. Comparison of the prediction by 27 different factors of coronary heart disease and death in men and women of the Scottish heart health study. British Medical Journal (1997); 315:722-729.

Tuomilehto J, Jousilahti P, Rastenyte D, Moltchanov V, Tanskanen A, Pietinen P, Nissinen A. Urinary sodium excretion and cardiovascular mortality in Finland: a prospective study. Lancet 357[9259], 848-51. 2001.

Valkonen VP, Voutilainen S, Myyssonen et al. Sodium and potassium excretion and the risk of acute myocardial infarction. Circulation 1998; 98 (Suppl 1):I-374(no.1962)

Vartianinen E, Puska P, Pekkanen J, Tuomilehto J, Jousilahti P. Changes in Risk Factors explain changes in mortality from ischaemic heart disease in Finland. British Medical Journal 1994; 309:23-7.

Vartianinen E, Sarti C, Tuomilehto J, Kuulasmaa K. Do changes in cardiovascular risk factors explain changes in mortality from stoke in Finland. British Medical Journal 1994; 310:901-4.

Vollmer WM, Sacks FM, Ard J, Appel LJ et al. Effects of diet and sodium intake on blood pressure: subgroup analysis of the DASH-Sodium trial. Annals of Internal Medicine 2001; 135:1019-1028.

Vollmer WM, Sacks FM, Svetkey LP. New insights into the effects on blood pressure of diets low in salt and high in fruits and vegetables and low-fat dairy products. Current Control Trials in Cardiovascular Medicine 2001; 2:71-74.

Watson RL, Langford HG, Abernethy J, Barnes TY, Watson MJ. Urinary electrolytes, body weight, and blood pressure. Pooled cross- sectional results among four groups of adolescent females. Hypertension 1980;2:93-8.

Watt GCM. Does salt sensitivity exist? Klinische Wochenschrift 1991; 69[Suppl XXV]:30-35.

Weil J, Bidlingmaier F, Dohlemann C, Kuhnle U, Strom T, Lang RE. Comparison of plasma atrial natriuretic peptide levels in healthy children from birth to adolescence and in children with cardiac diseases. Pediatric Research 1986;20:1328-31.

Weinberger MH, Miller JZ, Luft PC, Grim CE, Fineberg NS. Definitions and characteristics of sodium sensitivity and blood pressure resistance. Hypertension 1986; 8[suppl II]:II 127-II 134.

Weinberger MH, Finberg NS. Sodium and volume sensitivity of blood pressure: age and pressure change over time. Hypertension 1991; 18:67-71.

Weinberger MH. Salt sensitivity of blood pressure in humans. Hypertension 1996; 27(part 2):481-490.

Weinberger MH, Fineberg NS, Fineberg SE, Weinberger M. Salt sensitivity, pulse pressure, and death in normal and hypertensive humans. Hypertension 2001; 37[2]: 429-32.

Wheelock V, Hobbiss A. All you ever wanted to know about salt but were afraid to ask. Verner Wheelock Associates. Skipton, Yorkshire 1999.

Whelton PK, He J, Cutler JA, Brancati FL, Appel LJ, Follmann D, Klag MJ. Effects of oral potassium on blood pressure: meta-analysis of randomized controlled clinical trials. Journal of American Medical Association 1997; 277:1624-1632.

Whelton PK, Appel LJ, Espeland MA, et al. Sodium reduction and weight loss in the treatment of hypertension in older persons: a randomised controlled trial of nonpharmacologic interventions in the elderly (TONE): TONE Collaborative Research Group. Journal of the American Medical Association 1998; 279:839-846.

Whelton SP, Chin A, Xin X, He J. Effect of aerobic exercise on blood pressure: A meta-analysis of randomized, controlled trials. Annals of Internal Medicine 2002; 136:493-503.

Whitten CF. Metabolic data on the handling of NaCl by infants. Journal of Pediatrics 1969; 74(5):819-820.

Wilson AC, Forsyth JS, Greene SA, Irvine L, Hau C. Relation of infant diet to childhood health: seven year follow up of cohort of children in Dundee infant feeding study. British Medical Journal 1998; 316:21-5.

Wilson DK, Bayer L, Krishnamoorthy JS, Ampey-Thornhill G, Nicholson SC, Sica DA. The prevalence of salt sensitivity in an African-American adolescent population. Ethnicity and Disease 1999; 9(3):350-8.

Wu Y, Cai R, Zu B, Xu X. Effects of genetic factors and dietary electrolytes on blood pressure of rural secondary school students in Hanzhong. Hin Med Sci J 1991;6:148-152. Chinese Medical Science Journal 1991; 6:148-152.

Xin X, He J, Frontini MG, Ogden LG, Motsamai OI, Whelton PK. Effects of alcohol reduction on blood pressure: a meta-analysis of randomised controlled trials. Hypertension 2001; 38(5):1112-7.

Yamori Y, Nara Y, Mizushima S, Sawamura M, Horie R. Nutritional factors for stroke and major cardiovascular diseases: international epidemiological comparison of dietary prevention. Health reports (1994); 6:22-27.

Zhu K, He S, Pan X, Zheng X, Gu Y. The relation of urinary cations to blood pressure in boys aged seven to eight years. American Journal of Epidemiology 1987. 126:658-663.

Zoccali C, Mallamaci F, Cuzzola F, Leonardis D. Reproducibility of the response to short-term low salt intake in essential hypertension. Journal of Hypertension 1996; 14:1455-1459.

Annex 3

Main Sources of Sodium from Foods

Table 1: Amount of sodium and percentage contributions that different foods make to average intake of sodium/person/day (National Food Survey*)

Food	Sodium (g)	Salt (g)	% Contribution
Cereals & cereal products (e.g. bread, breakfast cereals, biscuits, cakes, pastries)	0.98	2.50	37.7
Meat & meat products	0.54	1.38	20.8
Other foods (e.g. soups, pickles, sauces, baked beans)	0.33	0.84	12.7
Processed vegetables (including crisps & snacks)	0.22	0.56	8.5
Milk & cream	0.14	0.36	5.4
Fats & oils	0.12	0.31	4.6
Cheese	0.11	0.28	4.2
Fish	0.07	0.18	2.7
Eggs	0.02	0.05	0.8
Fresh vegetables	0.02	0.05	0.8
Fruit	0.01	0.03	0.4
TOTAL	2.56	6.54	98.6

(1g sodium is equivalent to 2.55g salt)

* Sodium intakes for the National Food Survey are assessed from household food only and exclude salt added at the table or during preparation/cooking of food. Also excludes sodium in foods eaten out of the home.

Table 2: Amount of sodium and percentage contribution of food types to the average daily intake of sodium by age for boys (1997 National Diet and Nutrition Survey: young people aged 4-18 years*)

FOOD	Age in years 4-6 Sodium (g)	4-6 Salt (g)	4-6 %	7-10 Sodium (g)	7-10 Salt (g)	7-10 %	11-14 Sodium (g)	11-14 Salt (g)	11-14 %	15-18 Sodium (g)	15-18 Salt (g)	15-18 %
Cereals & cereal products	0.83	2.11	40	1.01	2.57	42	1.07	2.74	40	1.24	3.16	38
Meat & meat products	0.41	1.06	20	0.50	1.29	21	0.64	1.64	24	0.91	2.33	28
Savoury snacks	0.14	0.37	7	0.17	0.43	7	0.16	0.41	6	0.13	0.33	4
Vegetables & potatoes	0.21	0.53	10	0.17	0.43	7	0.24	0.62	9	0.29	0.75	9
Other foods (e.g. soups, pickles, sauces, baked beans)	0.08	0.21	4	0.12	0.31	5	0.13	0.34	5	0.20	0.50	6
Milk & milk products (excl cheese)	0.12	0.32	6	0.12	0.31	5	0.13	0.34	5	0.13	0.33	4
Cheese	0.06	0.16	3	0.07	0.18	3	0.05	0.14	2	0.10	0.25	3
Fats & spreads	0.04	0.11	2	0.07	0.18	3	0.08	0.21	3	0.07	0.17	2
Fish & fish dishes	0.06	0.16	3	0.05	0.12	2	0.05	0.14	2	0.07	0.17	2
Sugars, preserves, confectionery	0.02	0.05	1	0.05	0.12	2	0.05	0.14	2	0.03	0.08	1
Eggs & egg dishes	0.02	0.05	1	0.02	0.06	1	0.03	0.07	1	0.03	0.08	1
Drinks	0.04	0.11	2	0.02	0.06	1	0.03	0.07	1	0.07	0.17	2
Fruit & nuts	0.00	0.00	0	0.00	0.00	0	0.00	0.00	0	0.00	0.00	0
TOTAL (average daily intake)	2.07	5.28	99	2.40	6.12	99	2.68	6.84	100	3.27	8.33	100

*Sodium intakes for the National Diet and Nutrition Surveys exclude salt added at the table or during preparation/cooking of food.

Table 3: Amount of sodium and percentage contribution of food types to the average daily intake of sodium by age for girls (1997 National Diet and Nutrition Survey: young people aged 4-18 years*)

FOOD	4-6 Sodium (g)	4-6 Salt (g)	4-6 %	7-10 Sodium (g)	7-10 Salt (g)	7-10 %	11-14 Sodium (g)	11-14 Salt (g)	11-14 %	15-18 Sodium (g)	15-18 Salt (g)	15-18 %
Cereals & cereal products	0.72	1.85	39	0.91	2.31	42	1.02	2.60	38	1.21	3.08	37
Meat & meat products	0.35	0.90	19	0.45	1.15	21	0.59	1.51	22	0.69	1.75	21
Savoury snacks	0.15	0.38	8	0.17	0.44	8	0.21	0.55	8	0.16	0.42	5
Vegetables & potatoes	0.15	0.38	8	0.13	0.33	6	0.21	0.55	8	0.33	0.83	10
Other foods (e.g. soups, pickles, sauces, baked beans)	0.09	0.24	5	0.11	0.27	5	0.19	0.48	7	0.29	0.75	9
Milk & milk products (excl cheese)	0.11	0.28	6	0.11	0.27	5	0.11	0.27	4	0.10	0.25	3
Cheese	0.07	0.19	4	0.06	0.16	3	0.08	0.21	3	0.13	0.33	4
Fats & spreads	0.06	0.14	3	0.06	0.16	3	0.08	0.21	3	0.10	0.25	3
Fish and fish dishes	0.06	0.14	3	0.04	0.11	2	0.05	0.14	2	0.10	0.25	3
Sugars, preserves, confectionery	0.02	0.05	1	0.04	0.11	2	0.05	0.14	2	0.03	0.08	1
Eggs & egg dishes	0.02	0.05	1	0.02	0.05	1	0.03	0.07	1	0.07	0.17	2
Drinks	0.04	0.09	2	0.02	0.05	1	0.03	0.07	1	0.07	0.17	2
Fruit & nuts	0.00	0.00	0	0.00	0.00	0	0.00	0.00	0	0.00	0.00	0
TOTAL (average daily intake)	1.86	4.74	99	2.16	5.50	99	2.27	5.79	100	2.28	5.81	100

*Sodium intakes for the National Diet and Nutrition Surveys exclude salt added at the table or during preparation/cooking of food.

Annex 4

Dietary Reference Values for Sodium

The Dietary Reference Values (DRVs) for essential nutrients agreed by COMA[1] (DH, 1991) set a range of intakes based on assessment of the distribution of requirements for each nutrient. The Reference Nutrient Intake (RNI) represents the intakes required to meet 97.5% of the population. The Lower Reference Nutrient Intake (LNRI) represents the lowest intakes which will meet the needs of only 2.5% of the population.

DRVs for sodium were based on consumption patterns and the balance of risks and benefits which might practically be expected to occur, given the prevailing socio-cultural environment. It was difficult to determine a toxic threshold for sodium intake because a proportion of the population may be more susceptible to the effects of sodium than others (genetics, age and ethnic group may be factors).

Dietary Reference Values for Sodium mmol/d (mg/d)

AGE	LRNI	RNI
0-3 months	6 (140)	9 (210)
4-6 months	6 (140)	12 (280)
7-9 months	9 (200)	14 (320)
10-12 months	9 (200)	15 (350)
1-3 years	9 (200)	22 (500)
4-6 years	12 (280)	30 (700)
7-10 years	15 (350)	50 (1200)
11-14 years	20 (460)	70 (1600)
15-18 years	25 (575)	70 (1600)
19-50 years	25 (575)	70 (1600)
50+ years	25 (575)	70 (1600)

1mmol = 23 mg sodium; 1g salt contains 17.1 mmol sodium

1 Committee on Medical Aspects of Food and Nutrition Policy

Annex 5

Average Blood Pressures (mm Hg) for Men and Women in England, Scotland, and Northern Ireland

(Measurements based on a valid blood pressure reading)

COUNTRY*	AGE (years)							
		16-24	25-34	35-44	45-54	55-64	65-74	75+
England (2001)								
Men	Systolic	130	130	130	136	142	145	148
	Diastolic	64	71	76	81	82	79	77
Women	Systolic	120	120	123	132	140	147	154
	Diastolic	63	68	71	74	75	75	75
Scotland (1998)								
Men	Systolic	125	128	128	134	141	145	-
	Diastolic	62	69	74	79	80	78	-
Women	Systolic	117	117	121	130	139	149	-
	Diastolic	62	66	70	73	74	73	-
Northern Ireland (1997)								
Men	Systolic	125	130	131	131	143	144	148
	Diastolic	60	69	76	78	82	78	74
Women	Systolic	118	118	117	128	137	144	152
	Diastolic	62	66	68	72	73	74	73

* Data for Wales were unavailable

Annex 6

Overview of Sodium Metabolism and Regulation

Body sodium content is tightly regulated and closely related to water homeostasis. The total body content of sodium is regulated by a balance between dietary intake and renal excretion. Sodium excretion can be adjusted widely to match sodium intake and is highly efficient and adaptable. Changes in total body content of sodium are paralleled by changes in the extra cellular fluid (ECF) volume. When total sodium content is low, ECF volume is depleted and this is sensed by pressure receptors located in the cardiac atria and thoracic veins, which results in increased renal sodium conservation. When the total sodium content is high, volume overload develops which is sensed by high-pressure receptors in the carotid sinus and the renal juxtaglomerular apparatus, leading to an increase in natriuresis so that volume can be adjusted to normal.

The renin-angiotensin-aldosterone pathway is found in several different tissues, but most notably the kidney. The system regulates blood volume, arterial pressure, and cardiac and vascular function. Sympathetic stimulation, renal hypotension and reduced sodium delivery to the distal renal tubules generates renin release by the kidney. Renin acts on angiotensinogen to convert it to angiotensin I. Angiotensin converting enzyme (ACE), which is located in the pulmonary capillaries, cleaves angiotensin I to produce angiotensin II, a potent vasoconstrictor, which causes an increase in vascular resistance and hence arterial pressure.

Angiotensin II also acts on the adrenal cortex to produce aldosterone causing the kidneys to increase sodium and fluid retention; it also stimulates the release of antidiuretic hormone, which increases fluid retention.

A number of natriuretic factors increase renal sodium excretion. These include a specific natriuretic hormone, parathormone, prostaglandins and kinins. They exert their effects on the renal vasculature or on renal tubular reabsorption. Atrial natriuretic peptides (ANP), found in cardiac atrial tissue, appear to play an important role in the regulation of ECF volume, sodium metabolism, and blood pressure.

Human neonates are in negative sodium balance for the first four or so days of life and then gradually shift to positive sodium balance over 2-3 weeks. The renin-angiotensin-aldosterone system is known to be very active in the early postnatal phase. A slight increase in plasma renin activity occurs at 3-5 days of postnatal life followed by a marked decline in the next 1-6 weeks. By 3-5 years, plasma renin activity and plasma aldosterone values are similar to those of adults.

Annex 7

Sodium Sensitivity: Methods and Criteria[2]

Author	Protocol	Subjects	Criteria	Prevalence NT	HT
Kawasaki, 1978	109 meq Na (7days), 9meq Na (7 days), 240 meq Na (7days)	HT	ΔMean BP>10%	–	50%
Sullivan,1980	Ad libitum (1day), 10meq Na (4 days), ad libitum (2 days) 200meq Na (4days)	NT and BHT	ΔMean BP>5%	15%	29%
Fujita, 1980	9 meq Na (7 days), 249 meq Na (7 days), 9 meq Na (4 days) 40 mg furosemide t.i.d (1 day)	HT	ΔMean BP>10%	–	50%
Takeshita, 1982	70 meq Na (7days), 345 meq Na (7 days)	HT	ΔMean BP>10%	–	47%
Koomans, 1982	20-40 meq Na, 500 meq/100 ml CCr (until in balance)	CRF	ΔMean BP*	–	–
Campese, 1982	10meq Na (7 days), 100meq Na (7 days), 200 meq Na (7 days); random order	HT	ΔMean BP>10%	–	60%
Ishii, 1983	6g NaCl(2 days), 15g NaCl (5days)	NT and HT	ΔMean BP*	–	–
Koolen, 1983	50 meq Na (14 days), 300meq Na (14 days); random order	HT	ΔMean BP>10mm Hg	–	32%
Fujita, 1984	Ad libitum, mefruside 25 mg/day (7days), 180 meq Na (7days)	NT and BHT	ΔMean BP*	–	–
Weinberger, 1986	2l NS (4hr), 10meq Na, 40 mg furosemide t.i.d.	NT and HT	ΔMean BP↓>10mm Hg	26%	51%
Dustan and Kirk, 1988	I:150meq NA (3days), 9 meq Na, 1mg/kg furosemide (4 days). 25ml/kg NS (3days) II: 150meq NA (3days), 25ml/kg NS (3days), 9meq Na 1mg/kg furosemide (4days)	NT and HT	ΔMean BP*	–	–

Author	Protocol	Subjects	Criteria	Prevalence NT	HT
Sowers, 1988	40 meq Na (14 days), 180 meq Na (14 days)	NT and HT blacks	ΔMean BP>5% or systolic BP>10%	–	–
Rocchini, 1989	250 meq Na (14 days), 30 meq Na (14 days)	NT and obese	ΔMean BP*	–	–
Oshima, 1989	3g NaCl (7 days), 20g NaCl (7days)	Mild and moderate HT	ΔMean BP*	–	–
Sharma, 1989	220meq Na (7days), 20 meq Na (7days)	NT	ΔMean BP>3mm Hg	46%	–
Umeda, 1989	34meq Na(8days), 340 meq Na (8days)	HT	ΔMean BP>10%	–	–

BP, blood pressure; NS, normal saline; NT, normotensive; HT, hypertensive; BHT, borderline hypertensive; CRF, chronic renal failure.
* No numerical cutoff was used
Δ change

2 Source: Sullivan (1991)

Annex 8

Design of Studies since 1994 Examining the Effects of Salt and Blood Pressure on Morbidity and Mortality

Study	Type	Duration	Participants	Outcome of interest	Method for measurement of exposure	BP (mm Hg) criteria for hypertension SBP/DBP	Allowance for other cardiovascular risk factors in the analysis*
Alderman et al (1995) *Low urinary sodium is associated with greater risk of myocardial infarction among treated hypertensive men*	Prospective	3.5 years	Hypertensives (n=2937)	Morbidity and mortality events – incidence of MI, stroke, and CVD	Single 24-hour urine collection at baseline	160/90	Age Race Sex Smoking status CVD history Cholesterol levels
Alderman et al (1998) *Dietary sodium intake and mortality: the national health and nutrition examination survey (NHANES I)*	Prospective	17-21 years	General population (16% hypertensives) (n=11 346)	All-cause and CVD mortality	Single 24-hour dietary recall	160/95	Sex Age Race BMI CVD history Hypertension history

Study	Type	Duration	Participants	Outcome of interest	Method for measurement of exposure	BP (mm Hg) criteria for hypertension SBP/DBP	Allowance for other cardiovascular risk factors in the analysis*
Appel et al (1997) *A clinical trial of the effects of dietary patterns on blood pressure. DASH collaborative research group*	Randomised controlled trial	8 weeks	Normotensives & hypertensives (n= 459) age: ≥ 22y BP <160/80-95	Blood pressure	24-hour urine prior to intervention & during last 2 weeks of intervention	140/90	Sex Age Ethnicity Alcohol intake Physical activity BMI BP history Recent cardiovascular event
Cappuccio et al (1997) *Double-blind randomised trial of modest salt restriction in older people*	Randomised controlled trial	2 months	Hypertensive & normotensive untreated elderly subjects (n=47) age: 60-78y mean age: 66.8y BP range 123-205/64-112	Blood pressure	2 consecutive 24-hour urine collections at baseline, 2 weeks after salt restriction phase & end of each month of intervention	not stated	Age Sex CVD history Hypertension
Denton et al (1995) *The effect of increased salt intake on blood pressure of chimpanzees*	Randomised controlled trial	20 months	Chimpanzees (n=26) age: 5-18y	Blood pressure	24-hour urine collections by catheterisation	n/a	Age Sex

Study	Type	Duration	Participants	Outcome of interest	Method for measurement of exposure	BP (mm Hg) criteria for hypertension SBP/DBP	Allowance for other cardiovascular risk factors in the analysis*
Geleijnse et al (1996) *Long-term effects of neonatal sodium restriction on blood pressure*	Prospective	15 years	Children 15y of age followed up since birth (n=167)	Blood pressure	One overnight urine sample	n/a	Sex BMI Hypertension family history Smoking status Physical activity Alcohol intake
He et al (1999) *Dietary sodium intake and subsequent risk of cardiovascular disease in overweight adults*	Prospective	17-21 years	General population (n=9585)	Incidence and mortality of cardiovascular disease	Single 24-hour dietary recall at baseline and questioned whether always used table salt	160/95	Sex Age Race BMI Physical activity Hypertension Alcohol intake Smoking status Serum cholesterol CVD History

Study	Type	Duration	Participants	Outcome of interest	Method for measurement of exposure	BP (mm Hg) criteria for hypertension SBP/DBP	Allowance for other cardiovascular risk factors in the analysis*
Liebson et al (1995) *Comparison of five antihypertensive monotherapies and placebo for change in left ventricular mass in patients receiving nutritional-hygienic therapy in the treatment of mild hypertension study (TOMHS)*	Randomised controlled trial	4 years	Hypertensives (n=844) mean age: 55y	Change in left ventricular mass	2 consecutive overnight collections before randomisation and every 6 months thereafter Food records every 6 months	not stated	Age Sex Race BMI Alcohol intake Smoking status Physical activity History of hypertension Cholesterol levels History or clinical evidence of CVD
Morimoto et al (1997) *Sodium sensitivity and cardiovascular events in patients with essential hypertension*	Retrospective	7.3 years	Hypertensives (n=156)	Cardiovascular events	Urinary sodium excretion rate over last 3 days of each diet	not clear	Age Sex BMI Smoking status Serum cholesterol Blood pressure CVD history

Study	Type	Duration	Participants	Outcome of interest	Method for measurement of exposure	BP (mm Hg) criteria for hypertension SBP/DBP	Allowance for other cardiovascular risk factors in the analysis*
Sacks et al (2001) *Effects on blood pressure of reduced dietary sodium and the Dietary Approaches to Stop Hypertension (DASH) diet*	Randomised controlled trial	30 days	Normotensives & hypertensives (n=412) age: ≥ 22y BP range 120-159/80-95	Blood Pressure	24-hour urine during screening period and last week of intervention period	140-159/90-95	Sex Age Ethnicity Hypertensive status BMI CVD history Alcohol intake
Trials of Hypertension Prevention Collaborative Research Group (1997) *Effects of weight loss and sodium reduction intervention on blood pressure and hypertension incidence in overweight people with high normal blood pressure*	Randomised controlled trial	36-48 months	Healthy, moderately overweight men & women (n=2382) mean age: 44y	Blood pressure	At 6 months, 24-hour urine collection from 25% random sample At 18 & 36 months, 24-hour urine collection from all participants. 24-hour dietary recall & 3 day food record information	140/90	Sex Ethnicity BMI Smoking status Alcohol intake CVD history Current hypertension

Study	Type	Duration	Participants	Outcome of interest	Method for measurement of exposure	BP (mm Hg) criteria for hypertension SBP/DBP	Allowance for other cardiovascular risk factors in the analysis*
Tunstall-Pedoe et al (1997) *Comparison of the prediction by 27 different factors of coronary heart disease and death in men and women of the Scottish heart health study: cohort study*	Prospective	7.6 years	General population (n=11 629) age: 40-59y	Mortality from coronary heart disease, coronary events, coronary artery surgery, all-cause mortality	24-hour urine collection at baseline	n/a	Age Sex
Tuomilehto et al (2001) *Urinary sodium excretion and cardiovascular mortality in Finland: a prospective study*	Prospective	8-13 years	General population (n=2436) age: 25-64y	Frequency and mortality of cardiovascular disease and all-cause mortality	24-hour urine collection	n/a	Age Sex Serum cholesterol Blood pressure Smoking status BMI
Weinberger et al (2001) *Salt sensitivity, pulse pressure, and death in normal and hypertensive humans*	Prospective	27 years	Normotensives & hypertensives (n=708) age at baseline: 18-80y	Incidence and mortality caused by CVD events	Not carried out	not stated	Age Sex Race BMI Blood pressure

Study	Type	Duration	Participants	Outcome of interest	Method for measurement of exposure	BP (mm Hg) criteria for hypertension SBP/DBP	Allowance for other cardiovascular risk factors in the analysis*
Whelton et al (1998) Sodium reduction and weight loss in the treatment of hypertension in older persons. A randomized controlled trial of nonpharmacologic interventions in the elderly (TONE)	Randomised Controlled Trial	15-36 months	Treated hypertensives with BP<145/85 while receiving one anti-hypertensive drug (n=975) age: 60-80y mean age: 66.5y	Blood pressure Treatment with antihypertensive medication Cardiovascular events	24-hour urine collections & 24-hour dietary recall obtained twice during enrolment period, 9m, 18m & final visit	140/90	Age BMI Sex Race Smoking status Alcohol intake CVD history
Yamori et al (1994) Nutritional factors for stroke and major cardiovascular diseases: international epidemiological comparison of dietary prevention	Cross-sectional	n/a	General population (n = over 5000) age: 48-56y	Blood pressure Mortality rates for stroke and ischaemic heart disease	24-hour urine collection	not stated	Age Sex BMI Serum cholesterol

*Only main cardiovascular disease (CVD) risk factors of interest are listed: age, sex, alcohol intake, race, smoking status, body mass index (BMI), physical activity, hypertension/hypertension history (individual or family), CVD history (family or individual), cholesterol levels

Annex 9

Meta-Analyses & Systematic Reviews Published Since 1994 of Studies on Salt and Blood Pressure

Study	Inclusion criteria	Number of trials/participants/duration	Sodium excretion (mmol/24hr)	Mean change in SBP/DBP (mm Hg)
Alam et al (1999) *A meta-analysis of randomised controlled trials (RCT) among healthy normotensive and essential hypertensive elderly patients to determine the effect of high salt (NaCl) diet on blood pressure*	Randomised controlled trials of the effect of chronic salt ingestion in the elderly where BP and age data provided.	5 trials subjects 60y (n=158) 6 trials subjects close to 60y (n=318) (9 trials hypertensives/2 trials normotensives) mean duration 25 wks	Not stated	Pooled mean increase: Subjects 60y: 5.46/2.63 (CI: 3.56 to 7.36/1.18 to 4.08) Subjects close to 60y: 3.27/2.69 (CI: 1.23 to 5.31/1.44 to 3.94) All trials 5.58/3.5 (p=0.05/p=0.76)
Cutler et al (1997) *Randomised trials of sodium reduction: an overview*	Random allocation; free of confounding; sodium intake measured by 24h or 8h urinary sodium excretion; SBP, DBP or both measured; study subjects not pre-pubertal children; sodium intake goals within usual levels of industrialised countries.	22 trials hypertensives (n=946) median duration crossover trials 1m median duration parallel design 3m 12 trials normotensives (n=1689) median duration crossover trials 1m median duration parallel design 6m median/mean age of participants not stated	Median reductions: Hypertensives: crossover trials: 76 parallel design: 71 Normotensives: crossover trials 106 parallel design: 71	Pooled decrease: Hypertensives: 4.83/2.45 (CI: 3.79 to 5.87/1.77 to 3.13) Normotensives: 1.90/1.09 (CI: 1.18 to 2.62/0.61 to 1.57) All trials: 2.81/1.52 (CI: 2.23 to 3.39/1.14 to 1.9)

Study	Inclusion criteria	Number of trials/participants/duration	Sodium excretion (mmol/24hr)	Mean change in SBP/DBP (mm Hg)
Ebrahim & Davey Smith (1998) *Lowering blood pressure: a systematic review of sustained effects of non-pharmacological interventions*	Randomised controlled trials of blood pressure lowering by specific interventions – salt reduction, weight reduction, stress management, exercise, alcohol reduction; adults ≥ 40y; follow-up of ≥ 26 weeks	*salt reduction intervention:* 6 trials hypertensives (n=466) 2 trials normotensives (n=1095) mean/median trial duration not stated mean/median age of participants not stated	Not stated	Pooled decrease: Hypertensives: 2.9/2.1 (CI: 0 to 5.8/0.1 to 4.0) Normotensives: 1.3/0.8 (CI: 0.1 to 2.7/0.2 to 1.8)
Graudal et al (1998) *Effects of sodium restriction on blood pressure, renin, aldosterone, catecholamines, cholesterols, & triglyceride*	Random allocation to low or high sodium diet, sodium intake measured by 24-hour urine collection or from sample of at least 8hrs, SBP & DBP reported, mean age >15 years	58 trials hypertensives (n=2161) mean age 49y median duration 28 days 56 trials normotensives (n=2581) mean age 27y median duration 8 days	Mean difference between high and low sodium diets: Hypertensives 118 Normotensives 160	Pooled decrease Hypertensives: 3.9/1.9 (p<0.001/p<0.001) Normotensives: 1.2/0.26 (p<0.001/p=0.12)

Study	Inclusion criteria	Number of trials/participants/duration	Sodium excretion (mmol/24hr)	Mean change in SBP/DBP (mm Hg)
He and MacGregor (2002) *Effect of modest salt reduction on blood pressure. A meta-analysis of randomised trials. Implications for public health*	Randomised trials with a modest salt reduction in salt intake; no concomitant interventions; net reduction in urinary sodium intake $\geq$ 40 mmol; participants not children or pregnant Duration $\geq$ 4 weeks	17 trials hypertensives (n=734) median age 49y median duration 6 weeks 11 trials normotensives (n=2220) median age 49y median duration 4 weeks	Median decrease: Hypertensives: 78 Normotensives: 74	Pooled decrease: Hypertensives: 4.96/2.73 (p<0.001/0.001) Normotensives: 2.03/0.97 (p<0.001/0.001)
Hooper et al (2002) *Systematic review of long term effects of advice to reduce dietary salt in adults*	Randomisation adequate; usual or control dietary group; intervention aimed to reduce sodium intake & not multifactorial; participants not children/acutely ill/ pregnant/ institutionalised; follow-up at least 26 weeks; data on any of review outcomes available	5 trials untreated hypertensives (n=387) mean/median age not stated/range 16-64y 3 trials treated hyptertensives (n=801) mean/median age not stated/range 55-67y 3 trials normotensives (n=2326) mean age 40y median/mean trial duration not stated	6-12 months: 48.9 (CI 65.4-32.5) 13-60 months: 35.5 (CI 47.2-23.9)	Pooled decrease 6-12 months: 2.5/1.2 (CI: 3.8 to 1.2/1.8 to 0.7) 13-60 months: 1.1/0.6 (CI: 1.8 to 0.4/1.5 to −0.3)

Study	Inclusion criteria	Number of trials/participants/duration	Sodium excretion (mmol/24hr)	Mean change in SBP/DBP (mm Hg)
Midgley et al (1996) *Effects of reduced dietary sodium on blood pressure. A meta-analysis of randomised controlled trials*	Random allocation; dietary sodium intervention; measurement of urinary sodium excretion as measure of sodium intake; reporting of both SBP & DPB	28 trials hypertensives (n=1131) median age 47y median duration 29 days 28 trials normotensive (n=2374) median age 26y median duration 14 days	Mean excretion Hypertensives 95 Normotensives 125	Decrease per 100 mmol/d reduction in sodium excretion: Hypertensives: 3.7/0.9 (p<0.001/p=0.09) Normotensives: 1.0/0.1 (p<0.001/p=0.64)